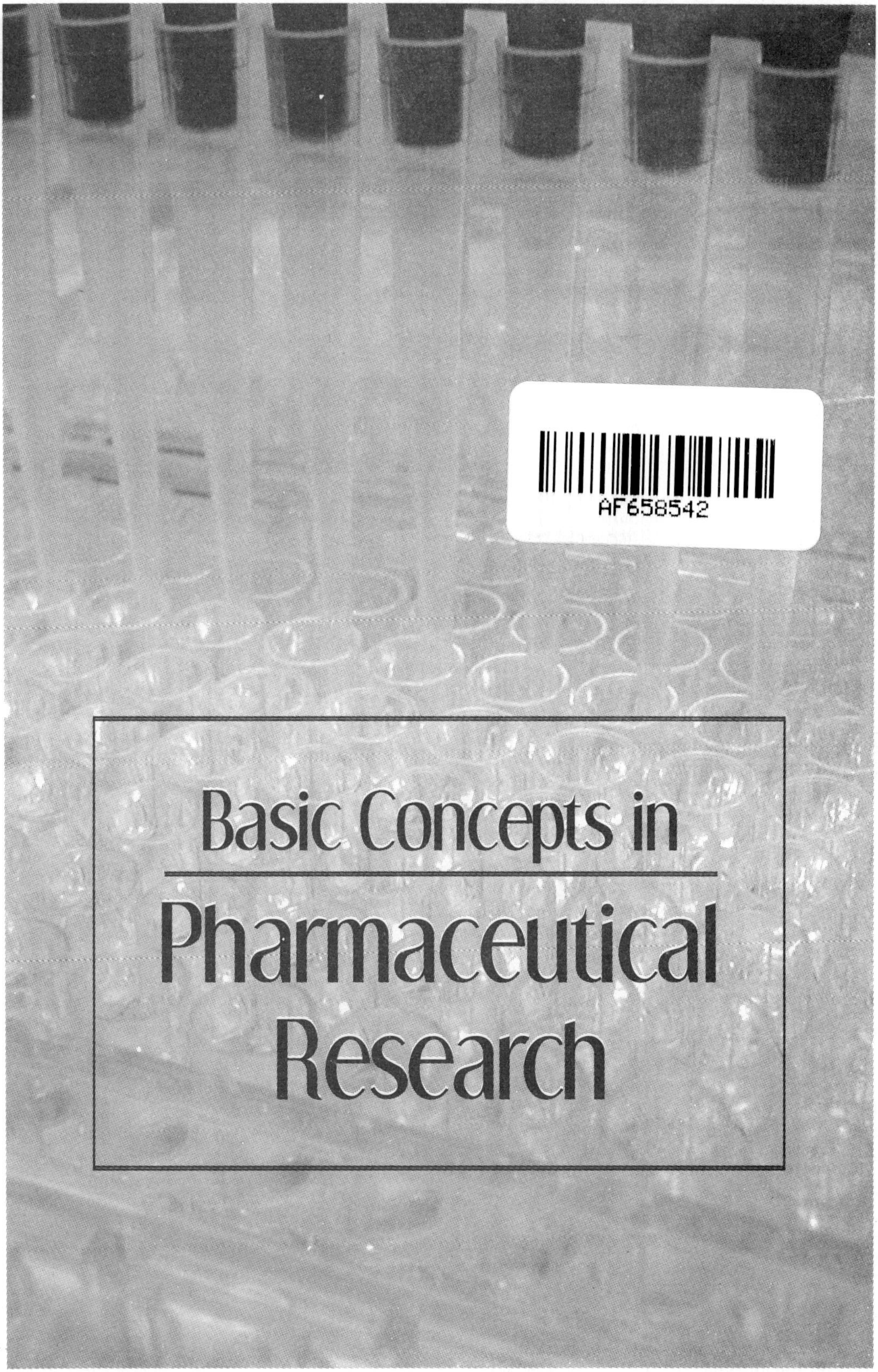

Basic Concepts in Pharmaceutical Research

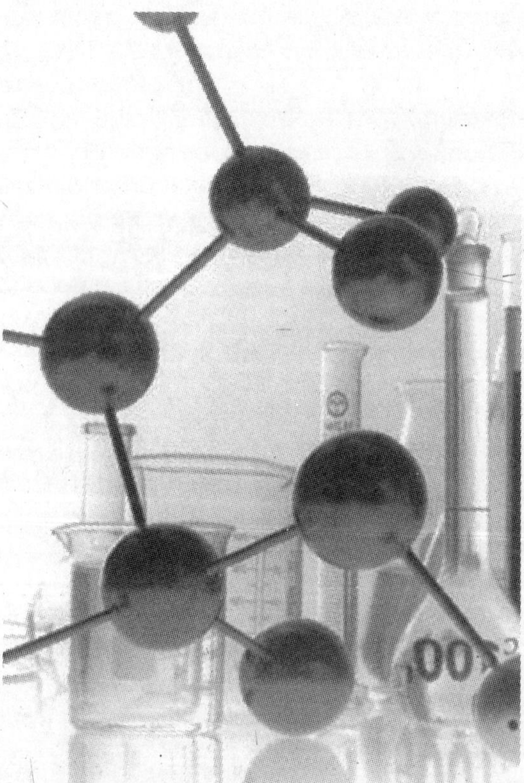

Basic Concepts in Pharmaceutical Research

Bijaya Ghosh PhD
Professor in Pharmaceutics
Department of Pharmaceutical Technology

Sonal Dubey PhD
Assistant Professor
Department of Pharmaceutical Chemistry

KLE University's College of Pharmacy
Rajajinagar, Bangalore, Karnataka

CBS

CBS Publishers & Distributors Pvt. Ltd.

New Delhi • Bengaluru • Chennai • Kochi • Kolkata • Mumbai
Hyderabad • Nagpur • Patna • Pune • Vijayawada

ISBN: 978-81-239-1815-0

First Edition: 2010
Reprint: 2014, 2017, 2019, 2020

Published by **Satish Kumar Jain** and produced by **Varun Jain** for
CBS Publishers & Distributors Pvt. Ltd.,
4819/XI Prahlad Street, 24 Ansari Road, Daryaganj, New Delhi - 110002
delhi@cbspd.com, cbspubs@airtelmail.in • www.cbspd.com
Ph.: 23289259, 23266861, 23266867 • Fax: 011-23243014

Corporate Office: 204 FIE, Industrial Area, Patparganj, Delhi - 110 092
Ph: 49344934 • Fax: 011-49344935
E-mail: publishing@cbspd.com • publicity@cbspd.com

Branches:
- ***Bengaluru:*** 2975, 17th Cross, K.R. Road, Bansankari 2nd Stage, Bengaluru - 70 • Ph: +91-80-26771678/79 • Fax: +91-80-26771680 E-mail: cbsbng@gmail.com, bangalore@cbspd.com
- ***Chennai:*** No. 7, Subbaraya Street, Shenoy Nagar, Chennai - 600030 Ph: +91-44-26681266, 26680620 • Fax: +91-44-42032115 E-mail: chennai@cbspd.com
- ***Kochi:*** Ashana House, 39/1904, A.M. Thomas Road, Valanjambalam, Ernakulum, Kochi • Ph: +91-484-4059061-65 Fax: +91-484-4059065 • E-mail: cochin@cbspd.com
- ***Kolkata:*** 6-B, Ground Floor, Rameshwar Shaw Road, Kolkata - 700014 Ph: +91-33-22891126/7/8 • E-mail: kolkata@cbspd.com
- ***Mumbai:*** 83-C, Dr. E. Moses Road, Worli, Mumbai - 400018 Ph: +91-9833017933, 022-24902340/41 • E-mail: mumbai@cbspd.com

Representatives:
- Hyderabad: 0-9885175004
- Patna: 0-9334159340
- Jharkhand: 0-9811541605
- Nagpur: 0-9021734563
- Pune: 0-9623451994
- Uttarakhand: 0-9716462459

Printed at:
J.S. Offset Printers, Delhi (India)

Preface

We have aimed this book at the postgraduate students of pharmaceutical sciences. The book gives an introduction to all the major statistical and analytical methods, and recent thrust areas in pharmaceutical research.

The theme of the book is to present an uncomplicated explanation of these approaches. We have covered a wide range of topics in a relatively small amount of space by selecting what we consider to be most important points involved in each technique, working on the theory that it is better to grasp a few key points rather than a large number of facts which are best consulted when a particular problem with a technique arises. For an in-depth coverage of the topics the readers are advised to consult specialized books on the particular topic of interest.

Statistics has become an integral part of pharmaceutical research. Starting from drug discovery to the formulation design and clinical trials, the experimental results are needed to be validated statistically. Though the time consumed in complicated mathematical calculations have been taken care by the software, a basic understanding is needed for the choice and usage of these programs. As teachers, we have often noticed the students getting confused about the basic terms used in the software and are unable to choose between the various options given in it. So we felt a book that would introduce basic terminology as well as the rationale of the statistical methods commonly used in pharmacy would be helpful to the students.

Drug design on the basis of structure–activity relationship and docking studies is an important concept and is taught as a subject at the postgraduate and final year undergraduate level. The second part of the book deals with this rationale drug designing approaches like QSAR, pharmacophore, docking, low cost synthesis and testing methodologies.

Some of the common instrumentation techniques like UV, NMR and HPLC that are routinely used in pharmaceutical investigations have also been discussed in this book.

There are many people who deserve credit and thanks for this endeavour. We want to thank all our postgraduate students especially to Kushal Tarafdar who had painstakingly drawn all the figures and diagrams in the book, and to Mr Sushant Sarkar for design of the cover. We also like to thank our friends and colleagues Mrs Uma Patil, Dr Versha Parcha, Miss Urmi Chaurasia, Mrs S Vasanti and Prof (Dr) Dinesh for their constant support; and Prof (Dr) BG Desai for maintaining the creative academic environment in the Institute.

Without the cooperation of family nothing is possible, therefore, we take this opportunity to thank Jayant (Dr Bijaya's brother), Manish, Aryaman, Avani (Dr Sonal's husband, son and daughter, respectively) who had given their moral support and encouragement for completing this book.

Bijaya Ghosh
Sonal Dubey

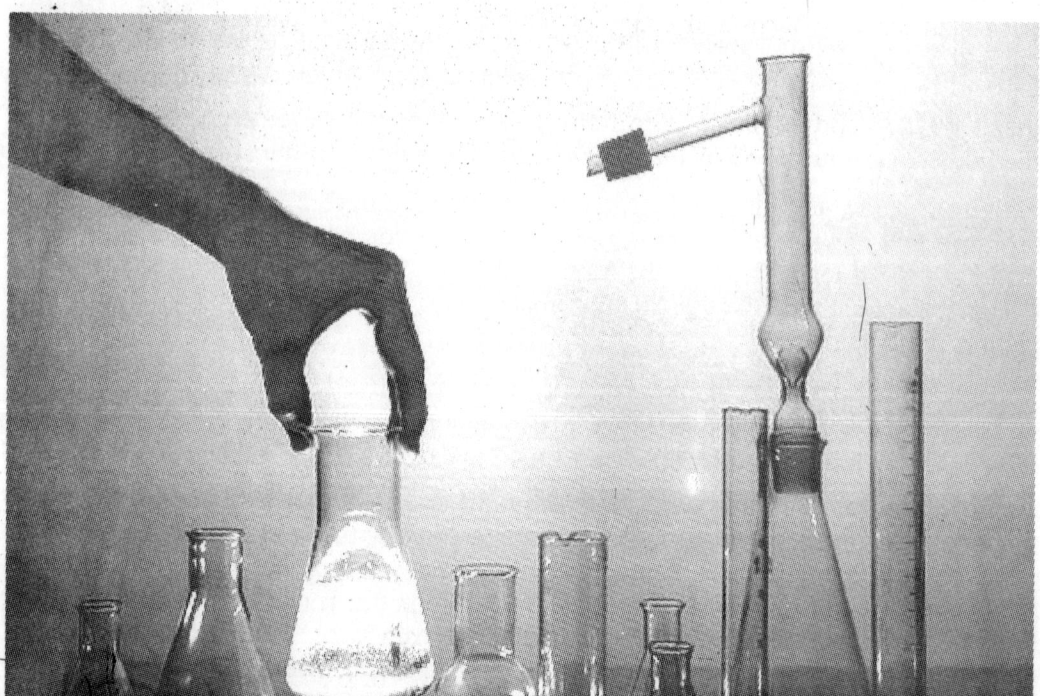

Contents

1 Basic Definitions and Probability Concepts

INTRODUCTION

Every subject has its vocabulary. In statistics too there are many terms that are used in everyday language. However, they have special meanings when used in the subject. Some terms such as *sample, range, population* and *deviation* would be used throughout the text. Hence it is necessary to know what these terms actually refer to in terms of statistics.

Variables

Values obtained from experiments are called *data. Variables are the characteristics or attributes of these data.* Data or variables can be of different types. They can be continuous variable or discrete variable.

Continuous Variable

A continuous variable can take on any value within a range, i.e. within a range it may have infinite number of possible values. The total *numbers* of possible values depend on sensitivity of the measuring device. For example, if a balance, capable of detecting the difference of 1 mg, is used for weighing 50 mg tablets in a weight variation test, weights may be shown as 49, 50 or 51 mg (3 values) but another balance that can measure up to the level of 0.1 mg can record much higher number of values. Suppose the tablet is actually 50.13 mg. The weight recorded in the second balance should be 50.1 mg. It will be unable to record the second digit after decimal as its sensitivity is up to 0.1 mg but at the same time it is much more efficient than the earlier balance as the total number of possible observations is much more. In a third balance which can record the difference of 0.01 mg, the total number of possible results is even larger. So the weight of a tablet is a continuous variable, which can take any value within a given range depending on the sensitivity of the measuring device used to record the weight.

Discrete Variable

A discrete variable can take on a countable number of values, i.e. within a range it may have a fixed number of possible values. Usually a discrete variable takes values, which are multiples of a certain value but not the values that lie within. For example, it is stated a variable X is an integral number in the range of 1–10. Here the possible number of values for *X* is just 10 (1, 2, 3, 4, 5, 6, 7, 8, 9, 10). *X* cannot have values like 1.5 or 1.25, etc. In pharmacy most of the data are discrete, e.g. number of anginal attacks or epileptic episodes suffered by a patient per week. Sometimes continuous variables can be ordered into the pattern of discrete data. For example, measuring headache in a continuous numerical scale is impossible. So it can be ordered as slight, moderate and severe headache in the three discrete classes.

Discrete data that are identified by names and can be categorized into classes are known as categorical variables or attributes. Tablets classified into two categories—defective and good, are an example of categorical or attribute type of variable.

So data can be classified as:

1. Continuous, e.g. blood sugar, weight.
2. Discrete associated with numbers, e.g. number of epileptic attacks per month.
3. Attributes: categorical which are ordered, e.g. degree of overweight.
4. Categorical non-ordered, e.g. adult, child.

Sample

Sample can be defined as relatively small number of observations taken from large populations. For example, after manufacturing, manufacturers need to evaluate whether the tablets have the required potency. But we cannot measure the potency of all tablets. So for determining the potency, a few tablets are taken from every batch as sample. To determine the statistical parameters accurately, sampling should be done with proper care according to predefined guidelines. Samples should be chosen in such a way that they represent the population.

Population

The total mass from where samples are chosen is called population. In the above case, total number of tablets in the batch is population. Similarly, all patients with a particular disease will be the population while patients whose parameters are to be measured are samples.

Parameter

Any measurable characteristic of the universe is called a parameter. In pharmaceutical evaluation of tablets, weight of the tablet is a parameter and disintegration time is another parameter. Greek letters are generally used to denote the parameters. Statistics usually characterizes a population by estimating its parameters.

Sample Statistic

Sample statistic is the values or results derived from sample. Usually statistics aims to derive the population parameters by evaluating samples. Sample statistic varies according to type, time and size of the sample. For example, if blood sugar of 5 diabetics is found to be 250, 300, 250, 300 and 400, the average blood sugar 300 is a sample statistic. But if the number of patients is increased to 10, some other values will be added. Say 200, 200, 200, 205, 115.5 are the values to be added. This will change the average to 242.05.

Average

Average is the sum of observations divided by number of observations. Average or mean is the most widely used statistical term. It is denoted by the symbol $\bar{X}$. In the above example the individual values were added and divided by the number of observations to find the average or mean value. Hence the average or $\bar{X} = 242.05$.

Median

Median is the value that divides the data into two halves. Hence median is the 50 percentile of a distribution. Suppose we have a set of 5 numbers 5, 7, 11, 17, 30.

Numerical mean is $(5 + 7 + 11 + 17 + 30)/5 = 14$ but the median will be the number 11, as 2 values 5 and 7 are lower than 11 and 2 values 17 and 30 are higher than 11. Median does not consider the value of the data. It is the midpoint value from which 50% of data are greater while 50% are lesser in value.

In percentile calculation, data are ranked in order of magnitude. The *n*th percentile denotes a value below which *n* percent of data are found. A rank of 90 percentile in an examination means the score is higher than that of 90% students or 90% of the students have scored below that particular student.

Mode

Mode is the value that occurs with the greatest frequency. Let us assume a data set of 9 values; 2, 5, 9, 7, 10, 7, 12, 7, 12. Here, out of 9 values, the value 7 occurs maximum number of times. All other values are less frequent than 7. So, the number 7 is the mode.

Range

In a given data set, range is the difference between the smallest and the largest value. If we have a data set of 1, 3, 5, 7, 9, 11, the range is 1 to 11.

Precision

Precision is a measure of variability; lesser the variability, greater is the precision. For determining an unknown parameter like disintegration time or potency of a tablet, experiments are repeated several times. The outcome obtained from these repeat experiments may vary and the result is expressed as mean of all the results. Let's suppose a tablet is assayed by two methods. Results obtained from the first method are 98, 100, 102 and mean is 100. The results from the second method are 96, 98, and 106 which also shows an average of 100. The extent of variability is more in the second method. Hence, it is less precise though the mean is same, i.e. 100 in both the methods.

Accuracy

Accuracy refers to the closeness of an individual observation to the true value. Let the real potency of a tablet be 100 mg. Two students are given the task of assaying the tablets.

The results obtained by the first student in 3 trials are 90, 90, 90 (mean 90) and that of second student are 100, 90, 95 (mean 95). Here the first student is more precise as his results have less variability (variability 0). The second student is closer to the true value and hence more accurate but less precise.

Bias

It is the tendency to find a result higher or lower than the true value. It may occur consciously (due to the preference for a particular result) or unconsciously (inaccurate methods).

Significant Figure

The number of significant figures in a measurement is equal to the number of digits that are known with some degree of confidence. Significant figures are critical when reporting scientific data because they give the reader an idea of how well we measure/report our data. As we improve the sensitivity of the equipment used to make a measurement, the number of significant figures increases (Table 1.1).

Table 1.1: Concept of significant figures

Dispensing balance	10 ± 1 g	1 significant figure
Chemical balance	1.1 ± 0.01 g	3 significant figures
Analytical balance	1.01 ± 0.001 g	4 significant figures

In statistics rounding should not be done before all calculations are complete. Significant figure should be reported with reasonable precision.

Variance

Variance is a measure of deviation from the mean value. It is expressed as

$$\sigma^2 = \frac{\Sigma\left(X-\overline{X}\right)^2}{N} \qquad \text{(Eq. 1.1)}$$

Here σ^2 represents true variance.

To clarify the concept let's take a set of values as 1, 3, 7, and 5. Here

mean = (1 + 3 + 7 + 5)/4 = 4.

Difference of the 1st value from mean is

(4 – 1) = 3 and the square of this difference is 9.

Difference of the 2nd value from mean is

(4 – 3) = 1 and the squared difference is 1.

Difference of the 3rd value from mean is

(4 – 7) = –3. The squared difference is 9.

Difference of the 4th value from mean is

(4 – 5) = –1 and squared difference is 1.

Sum of squares of difference of each value from mean, i.e.

$\Sigma(X-\overline{X})^2$ is (9 + 1 + 9 + 1) = 20.

Number of observations, i.e. number of values from which mean is obtained is denoted as N.

According to the above formula, the variance is 20/4 = 5 which is the true variance.

Here, we have dealt with a small set of numbers (4 values only) but in real life all the values of a population cannot be known. Hence, to get an unbiased estimate, we take variance on the upper side by dividing the sum of squared differences with $N - 1$.

Sometimes the use of $N - 1$ rather than N in the denominator confuses us. Actually, the use of $N - 1$ in place of N increases the value of variance slightly and makes the sample variance an unbiased estimate of the population variance (S^2).

$$S^2 = \frac{\Sigma\left(X - \overline{X}\right)^2}{N - 1} \qquad \text{(Eq. 1.2)}$$

Where, S^2 represents variance obtained from the sample.

Standard Deviation (S or s.d.)

Standard deviation is the square root of variance. In most of the calculators, there are two options for standard deviation; standard deviation for $N - 1$ and N. When the number of observations is less than the total population, the value of *s.d.* is calculated for $N - 1$.

If the number of observations is large (say greater than 30) the values obtained with N and $N - 1$ are practically same and *s.d.* can be obtained for N.

In the above example, standard deviation is

$$\sqrt{\frac{20}{3}} \text{ and } \sqrt{\frac{20}{4}}$$

i.e. 2.58 and 2.23 for $\sigma n-1$ and σn respectively. The mean along with standard deviation is a succinct description of data distribution or spread of data. The larger the magnitudes of standard deviation, more spread out the data are.

The symbol used for standard deviation is usually S but sometimes it is written as *s.d.* also. It is mathematically expressed as:

$$s.d. = \sqrt{\frac{\Sigma\left(X - \overline{X}\right)^2}{N - 1}} \qquad \text{(Eq. 1.3)}$$

Standard Error (SE)

Standard deviation of mean or error of mean is a measure of variability of mean. Results of pharmaceutical experiments are often expressed as mean ± standard error. Statistics shows standard deviation of mean is equal to standard deviation calculated from individual data divided by $\sqrt{N}$.

$$S_x = \frac{S}{\sqrt{N}} \qquad \text{(Eq. 1.4)}$$

Coefficient of Variation (CV)

Coefficient of variation is a measure of relative variation. $\bar{X}$ represents the mean of data set and standard deviation (S) is the measure of spread of the data. So $S/\bar{X}$ is the relative measure of variability and also known as relative standard deviation (RSD).

It can be expressed as percentage coefficient of variation too.

$$CV\% = (S/\bar{X}) \times 100 \quad \text{(Eq. 1.5)}$$

Biological experiments usually have high CV.

Coding

Statistical calculations are lengthy and time-consuming. But there are certain short cuts to simplify the calculations involving mean and standard deviations.

Rule 1: Adding or subtracting a constant to the individual values causes the mean to be increased and decreased by a constant but keeps the variance and s.d. unchanged.

For example, the mean of 2, 4, 6 is 4 and s.d. is 2.

If we add 50 to each of the values we get 52, 54, 56 and new mean is 54, which is 50 + 4 (old mean) but s.d. is unchanged, i.e. 2.

Rule 2: If the mean of a set of data is $\bar{X}$ and s.d. is S, multiplying or dividing each value by a constant k results in a new mean kX or X/k. Similarly, the new s.d. will be kS or S/k.

In the above example, the values are 2, 4 and 6. If each of the values is multiplied by 2 then data will be 4, 8 and 12.

This will result a mean of 8, i.e. (4 × 2) and s.d. of 4 (2 × 2).

By this rule, any data set can be converted to normalized data in which mean is zero and s.d. is 1. If a number equal to the value of mean is subtracted from each value of the data set, and is divided with standard deviation, the resultant data will have the mean of 0 and s.d. of 1.

CONCEPT OF PROBABILITY

Probability is the relative frequency with which an event occurs in nature. In statistics, it represents a measure of uncertainty to find a particular result. Often we come across situations in Pharmacy, where hypotheses or decisions are to be supported by the experimental results. However, the experimental results may be affected by many factors. Errors may be incorporated into the experiment due to faulty measurements, process deviations and personal variations. Hence data obtained from the experiments or epidemiological surveys are subjected to statistical analysis to find the probability of error. In statistics, probability is expressed with the symbol P. When we say $P < 0.05$, it indicates the chance of getting the result by mistake is only 5%. Exact probabilities are always unknown.

Statistical theories are based on normal distribution which indicates that if an experiment is repeated n times, the n numbers of results obtained would be symmetrically distributed around the mean. A particular result (i.e. mean) is likely to occur maximum number of times, (i.e. with the highest frequency) and results, which are higher or lower than mean, will have lesser frequency. In the mathematical term, the probability of a particular event is expressed as $P(A)$. The following assumptions are used to calculate the probability value.

1. $0 \le P(A) \le 1$ (Eq. 1.6)

   0 is impossible event; probability of an experimental outcome cannot be less than 0, whereas 1 is a certain event.

2. $P(A \text{ or } B \text{ or } C\ldots) = P(A) + P(B) + P(C)$ (Eq. 1.7)

   The total chance of occurring A or B or C is the sum of the chances of occurrence of A, B and C, when A, B, C are mutually exclusive, i.e. when A occurs neither B nor C can occur or vice versa.

3. $P(A) + P(B) + P(C) = 1$ (Eq. 1.8)

   when A, B and C exhaust all possible outcome.

4. $P(A \text{ or } B) = P(A) + P(B) - P(A \text{ and } B)$ (Eq. 1.9)

   When two events A and B are not mutually exclusive, i.e. both A and B can occur simultaneously and $P(A \text{ or } B)$ indicates the probability of getting A or B alone.

5. $P(A \text{ and } B) = P(A \mid B)\, P(B)$ (Eq. 1.10)

   Here, $P(A \mid B)$ is known as the conditional probability of A given that B also occurs. Let's assume that in a quality control test of tablets, it was seen that 2/3rd of cracked tablets also become colorless. The probability of cracked tablets is 10% or 0.1 of the total tablets. Hence, 2/3rd of 0.1 or 0.066 is the probability of getting tablets with both the defects (both cracked and colorless).

6. $P(A \text{ and } B) = P(A) \cdot P(B)$ (Eq. 1.11)

   The above expression shows the probability of getting A and B together, when events are independent of each other. In our example only some 66% of the cracked tablets were colorless. No intact tablet was colorless and overall a small percentage 6.6% (2/3 of 10%) of the total tablets was colorless. If the condition, i.e. only cracked tablets can be colorless, is removed, the probability of getting tablets with both the defects will be much lesser $(0.1 \times 0.066) = 0.0066\%$.

Probability Distributions

Binomial Distribution

The method of probability calculation depends on the nature of data.

When a single observation can be dichotomized, i.e. can be placed in one of the two possible categories, binomial distribution can be used. It is applicable to experimental results that have only two possible outcomes; for example pass or fail, defective or good, right or wrong.

Since the outcome can only fall into only one or the other category, the sum of the two options is 1.

Let us assume the options are 'pass' or 'fail'.

So combined probabilities of success and failure, i.e. $P(\text{success}) + P(\text{failure}) = 1$.

The standard deviation of a binomial distribution with probability of success p in N trials is given by the expression $\sqrt{\frac{pq}{N}}$.

Since $p + q = 1$, q can be substituted by $1 - p$.

$$\text{Hence, s.d. of the } p \text{ (success)} = \sqrt{\frac{p(1-p)}{N}} \qquad \text{(Eq. 1.12)}$$

If the probability of passing is 75% and failing is 25%, then P (passing) = 0.75 and P (failing) = 0.25. Standard deviations of the actual outcome if the examination is conducted 16 times will be

$$\sqrt{\frac{0.75 \times 0.25}{16}} = 0.108.$$

This indicates that in reality the probability of passing may vary between 0.75 + 0.108 = 0.858 on the upside and 0.75 – 0.108 = 0.642 on the downside.

The probability of the outcome of a binomial experiment consisting of N trials can be computed from the expansion of the expression $(p + q)^n$ where p = success, q = failure.

If we toss a coin 2 times there may be only 3 outcomes:

1. 2 heads,
2. 2 tails,
3. 1 head and 1 tail.

The probability of occurring head and tail (p and q) are same. So head p = 0.5 and tail q = 0 .5. By expanding the equation we get,

$$(0.5 + 0.5)^2 = (0.5)^2 + 2 \times 0.5 \times 0.5 + (0.5)^2$$

In this expression

0.25 is the probability for both heads.

0.25 is the probability for both tails.

0.5 is the probability for getting 1 head and 1 tail.

Here total of all options is 1 and all options are exhausted.

In general, with N tossing, $N + 1$ type of results are possible. If the coin is tossed 3 times, 4 types of outcomes are possible. Here the outcomes are all 3 heads, all 3 tails, 2 head 1 tail and 1 head 2 tails. Similarly, in the binomial expression if n is assigned a value of 3 it will have 4 terms, which will represent all 4 options.

By definition $p + q = 1$

So whatever be the value of N the sum total would always be 1.

Probability of X successes in N trials

$$= \binom{N}{X} p^X q^{N-X} \qquad \text{(Eq. 1.13)}$$

Where, $$\binom{N}{X} = \frac{N!}{X!(N-X)!}$$

Suppose in a survey of blood groups, the chance of getting people with O+ve blood is 0.1. As there are only two options (a person is either O+ve or not) this distribution is binomial in nature. If we test 4 people there are 5 possibilities.

1. No one is O+ve.
2. 1 person is O+ve.
3. 2 people are O+ve.
4. 3 people are O+ve.
5. All people are O+ve.

Of these options the probability of any option can be calculated by the above equation.

For example, the probability of the 4th option, i.e chance of 3 of 4 people being O+ve, is given by

$$\frac{4\times3\times2\times1}{3\times2\times1}(0.1)^3(0.9) = 0.0036$$

N (number of people tested) = 4, X (probability of a particular option) = 3,
p = probability of natural occurrence = 0.1.
So, q or $1-p = 1-0.1 = 0.9$.

The Normal Distribution

It is the most familiar, symmetrical bell-shaped distribution curve. *In theoretical normal distribution, data points extend from positive infinity to negative infinity.* Like all other curves, this curve too has two axes. The independent variable (X) is represented in X axis while the ordinate or Y axis shows the frequency of occurrence of a particular value of X.

The function of normal probability density (Y) is defined as

$$Y = \frac{1}{\sigma\sqrt{2\pi}} e^{-(1/2)(X-\mu)^2/\sigma^2} \qquad \text{(Eq. 1.14)}$$

μ = mean
σ = standard deviation
X = value of the observation
e = base of natural logarithm 2.718...
Y = function of X, ordinate of the normal curve.

Note that, the two most important parameters that affect the value of Y are μ and σ.

As the individual values of X deviate from μ the value of $(X - \mu)^2$ increases. As the overall sign of the exponent is negative the value of Y decreases with increase of $(X - \mu)^2$. In real life also we see the farther the value of X from mean–its chance of occurring decreases exponentially.

Let's assume a set of values 2, 3, 5, 5, 5, 7, 8.

The mean and standard deviation are 5 and 2.08 respectively.

From Eq. 1.14 the chance of occurrence of a particular value 2 is found to be 0.067.

But the chance of occurrence of the value 4 is much higher, i.e. 0.17.

The normal distribution can be defined by two parameters—mean and standard deviation. If these parameters are known, the distribution can be reconstructed. There can be infinite number of normal distributions. All of them can be reconstructed if we know the mean and the measure of their spread, which is standard deviation. Areas under the normal curve represent probabilities, which are obtained by appropriate integration of the above equation.

Frequency Distribution Curve

Statistics handles large amount of data. Hence it has ways to present and arrange these data in concise and compact manner. Frequency distribution is the most popular way to present a data summary.

While making a frequency distribution curve, total amount of data are divided into certain class intervals. Frequency in each class is expressed as the number of observations (data) that comes under a particular class. Class intervals in frequency distribution curves are to be made according to judgment. Frequency represents the occurrence of an event in a particular class interval.

For example, body weight pattern of a class of 20 students is to be displayed in a pictorial manner.

It is observed body weights varied between 33 to 45 kg.

Here we can arrange the data in 3 intervals, 30–35, 35–40, and 40–45.

Let the weight recorded from individual students be, 32, 33, 32, 34, 36, 44, 45, 34, 34, 45, 32, 45, 38, 39, 41, 39, 37, 36, 32, 34.

The 1st interval (30–35 kg category) has 32, 33, 32, 34, 34, 34, 32, 32, 34, i.e. 9 values.

The 2nd interval (35–40 kg category) has 36, 38, 39, 39, 37, 36, i.e. 6 values.

In the 3rd interval (40–45 category) falls 5 body weights 44, 45, 45, 45, 41, i.e. 5 values.

These values 9, 6, and 5, belonging to the different intervals values are the frequencies of the respective categories in a frequency-distribution curve (Table 1.2, Fig. 1.1).

Table 1.2: Data arranged in a frequency-distribution pattern

Body weight	*Frequency*
30–35	9
35–40	6
40–45	5

Standard Normal Curve

Though there is infinite number of normal curves, the standard normal curve is the one extensively used in statistics. The standard normal curve has a mean of 0 and standard deviation of 1. Table 1.3 shows the cumulative areas under the standard normal curve. The shaded portion of the Fig. 1.2 indicates the areas enclosed between the values of infinity and Z.

Figure 1.2 shows when value of Z is –1.96 the area is 0.025, which indicates only 2.5% values will belong to the area enclosed–infinity and –1.96.

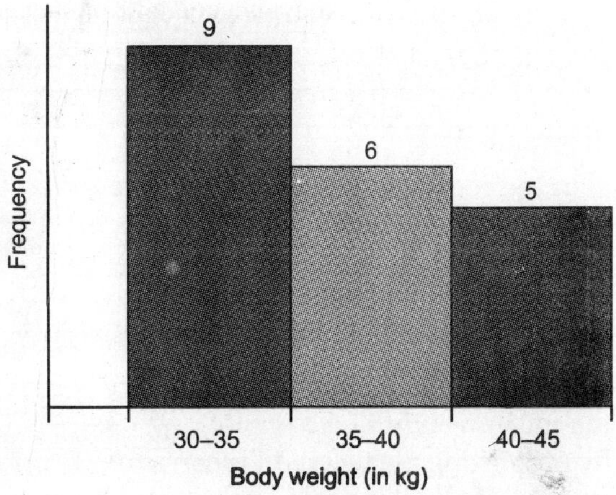

Fig. 1.1: A frequency-distribution curve (based on data from Table 1.2)

Table 1.3: Area between ± *Z* in standard normal distribution

Z	*Area between* ± Z
0.84	0.60
1.00	0.68
1.28	0.80
1.65	0.90
1.96	0.95
2.32	0.98
2.58	0.99

Conversion of Normal Curves to Standard Normal Curve

To find out the probability of occurrence of a particular value of X in a data set, we need to consult the area values for a standard normal curve. But the values of a real distribution are not in the form of standard normal curve. Hence, the first step of probability calculation is to convert the normal curve of mean μ and standard deviation σ to the corresponding standard normal curve of mean 0 and s.d. 1.

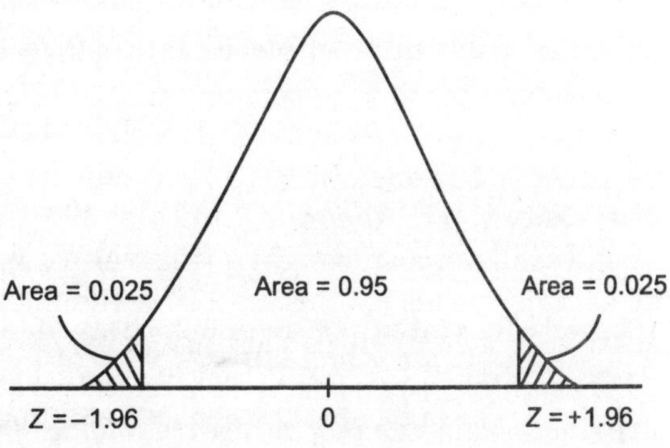

Fig. 1.2: Shape of normal curve

In standard normal curve, *Z* represents the value of independent variable. To have an idea of the conversion concept, take the example of a photographic frame. Standard normal curve has definite structure like the photographic frame. It has a mean of 0 and standard deviation of 1. If a photograph is smaller than the frame, it can be enlarged to fit the frame or reduced if the frame is small. Similarly, the real values of X in a normal curve can be transformed by a conversion factor to fit the standard normal distribution.

In the conversion process, X is converted to Z by the following equation.

$$Z = \frac{(X - \mu)}{\sigma} \qquad \text{(Eq. 1.15)}$$

Here Z of the standard normal curve is equivalent to X in the simple normal curve.

For example, let us take the case of weight variation of capsules. It was found that the mean weight of a batch of capsules is 250 mg and the standard deviation is 5 mg. By converting the values of mean and s.d. into standard normal curve, we can calculate fraction of tablets that is likely to be above or below a certain weight. For example, we want to know, what proportion of the capsules is likely to have a weight less than 255 mg?

To solve this problem, the values have to be substituted in Eq. 1.15.

First, we have to find the equivalent value of Z for 255 mg.

The equivalent value of Z obtained is (255 – 250)/5 = 1.

Next we have to consult the Z table (Appendix 1). Figure 1.2 extends from – infinity to + infinity, having a 0 in between. So, the capsule weights lesser than 255 mg will be represented on the left side of +1 mark and those of weight greater than 255 mg will be on the right side of +1 mark.

According to 1, the area between infinity and 1 is 0.68. So 68% capsules are likely to have weight lesser than 255 mg.

Central Limit Theorem

Central limit theorem is possibly the most important theorem in statistics. It discusses about the distribution of means rather than the distribution of individual values.

Consider a batch or population of 10,000,00 capsules. From it, we can take *n* batches of samples (say 60 capsules) and calculate the mean of every sample batch. If we repeat the process 10 times (n = 10), we will be getting 10 means each of which has 60 observations. The theorem indicates that if the original population, i.e. 10,000,00 capsules, has a mean weight μ (the true mean) and a variance of σ^2, the distribution of the sample means (in this case 10 means) tends to be normal around the population mean (true mean) with a variance of σ^2/N.

The point that makes this theorem important is that the original population may or may not have a normal distribution but means obtained from the samples will be normally distributed around the population mean provided the sample size is large.

This point allows any distribution irrespective of its nature to be treated by the rules of normal distribution. The only condition to be met is the use of 'a large sample size.' Even in asymmetric distribution like 1, 2, 3, 4 where data seem to have rising pattern, (i.e. a peak but no trough), if sample sizes are large (greater than 20) means are distributed around the population mean.

THE POISSON DISTRIBUTION

The Poisson distribution can be considered to be an approximation to the binomial distribution.

It has application in Pharmacy when the sample size is large. The probability of observing a defective item is often calculated using the Poisson ratio. For example, let us assume that a batch of injection was subjected to sterilization process and probability of having an unsterilized injection is to be calculated.

The probability of observing X events of a given type in N observations, where the probability of observing the event in a single observation is P (X), is expressed as

$$P(X) = \frac{\lambda^X e^{-\lambda}}{X!} \qquad \text{(Eq. 1.16)}$$

Where,

$\lambda = NP$

e = Base of natural logarithms (2.718)

N = Number of observations

We may use the Poisson distribution to compute the probability of finding one defective injection in a sample of 100 taken from a batch with 1% defective injection. Applying Eq. 1.16, we have $N = 100$ and $P = 0.01$. Hence $NP = (100)(0.01) = 1$, $X = 1$.

$$P(1) = \frac{(1)^1 e^{-1}}{1!} = 0.368$$

So, $P(1) = 0.368$

If the proportion of the defective tablet was higher, (e.g. 2%), the probability of getting only 1 defective item in a batch of 100, would be 0.27. Apparently, the result seems contradictory, but then we have to think the reverse way.

When we say the chance of getting 1 defective item in 100, it indicates 99 items should be defect-free. In a population of 2% defective items, the chance of getting of 99 non-defective item is lesser than with 1% defective items as is indicated by the calculated probability.

THE *t* DISTRIBUTION ('STUDENT'S *t*')

The *t* distribution is an extremely important probability distribution. This distribution is constructed by repeatedly taking samples of size *N* from a normal distribution and computing the sample mean and from it value of '*t*.'

The value of *t* is calculated from the equation

$$t = \frac{\overline{X} - \mu}{S/\sqrt{N}} \qquad \text{(Eq. 1.17)}$$

Where $\overline{X}$ is the sample mean, μ the true mean of the normal distribution, and *S* the sample standard deviation. The distribution of the *ts* is thus obtained from the *t* distribution. The exact shape of the *t* distribution depends on sample size (degrees of freedom), but the t distribution is symmetrically distributed about a mean of 0, as shown in the Fig. 1.3.

The concept of t distribution can be explained as follows. Let us take a population of tablets with mean weight of 100 and s.d. of 5 mg. Now let us take 100 samples from this population, each with a sample size of 4. For each batch of 4 samples, mean and s.d. are calculated. These values can be converted to t values using Eq. 1.18. Now, 100 *ts* obtained can be plotted as a histogram. It is seen that the distribution is symmetric around a mean of 0.

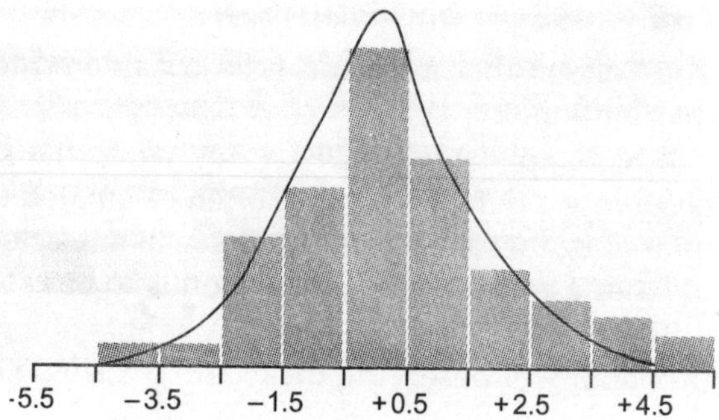

Fig. 1.3: The shape of a *t* distribution

F Distribution

F distribution is the ratio of two independent variance estimates obtained from the same normal distribution. This distribution is used to test the difference of means as well as to test the equality of two variances.

If the first sample contains N_1 observations and the second sample contains N_2 observations, the F distribution shows the ratio of variances of these two samples. F value is calculated as:

$$F = \frac{S_1^2}{S_2^2} \quad \text{(Eq. 1.18)}$$

BIBLIOGRAPHY

1. Daniel W Wayne: *Biostatistics: A Foundation for Analysis in Health Sciences*, Seventh edition, John Wiley and Sons, 1999.
2. De, Muth James E, Basic statistics and pharmaceutical statistical applications, Marcel Dekker, Inc, 1999.
3. Gurumani N: *An Introduction to Biostatistics*, Second edition, 2005.
4. Sanford Bolton, *Practical and Clinical Applications*, Third edition, Marcel Dekker, Inc, 1997.

2 Estimation and Hypothesis Testing

INTRODUCTION

One of the common practices of statistics is to estimate the parameters of a sample and come to a decision about the entire population from these sample parameters. Sampling is done in such a way that sample mean and sample variance can predict the population mean and population variance. 'Whether a finding is statistically significant or not?' is an important question in pharmaceutical research. 'The new formulation is superior to the existing formulations and difference is statistically significant at 1% level' is almost a general statement in the regulatory literature while introducing a new formulation or a new medicine. This chapter discusses some of the methods used for such estimation and decision-making.

Pharmaceutical statistics deals mainly with two types of problems.

1. Estimation of parameters like mean and standard deviation, which can describe the population.
2. Comparisons of groups/products where a new extract of a drug or a formulation is compared with other existing ones.

The first type deals with estimation while the second type is concerned with hypothesis testing.

CONCEPT OF ESTIMATION

What is Estimation?

The properties or parameters of the population are derived from the sample. However, more often than not, sample is a minute fraction of the total population. So there is always a chance that sample mean is not the real mean, but quite close to it. *Estimation methods deal with determining and reporting the parameters of the entire population by testing the samples, which are just a minute fraction of it.*

How the Estimated Parameters should be Reported?

Suppose the average age of people in a city is to be determined. Here, the sum total of every single person living in that city constitutes the population. But sampling will be done on a few hundreds and from this, a prediction would be made about the average

age and standard deviation of ages of people living in that city. But can the analysis of age of a few people correctly predict the age of the entire population? The answer is possibly 'No'. The chance of error is inbuilt in the system of analysis itself. Hence, while reporting the result of an experiment, (e.g. mean age), it is better to report a range rather than a single value.

What is Confidence Interval?

A confidence interval is the range within which the true mean lies.

In pharmacy, often we test the weight of a few tablets of a batch to make a statement about the mean tablet weight. The chance of error is ingrained in the method and accuracy of the result will depend on the number of units used for sampling. It is more accurate to say that the mean weight of a tablet is between a range rather than stating a single value with a certain degree of probability. Hence, it is usually reported as a confidence interval within which the true mean lies.

How the Confidence Interval is Determined?

Confidence interval is a range, expressed as mean ± SE of a certain value. The mean is the sample mean. However, the second part, i.e. ± SE determines width of the range. The value of this part depends upon the source of data and type of tests performed to determine the sample statistic. In general, the width of the range depends on the standard deviation and degree of certainty desired. If we want to be more confident or the level of certainty desired is high (say > 99%) we will have to specify a wider range. But the exact width of that range will depend on sample size and value of standard deviation. The crucial factor is standard deviation. If the standard deviation is known or given, we will select one method; if unknown we have to select another method.

Determination of Confidence Interval with Known Standard Deviation

Determination of true standard deviation needs assessment of all data in a population. Alternatively, it may be determined from historical data, i.e. the s.d. of many batches determined over a long period. A known standard deviation indicates decreased uncertainty. Confidence interval is expressed in percentage.

The formula is

$$P\%\ (\text{confidence interval}) = \bar{X} \pm \frac{Z_p \sigma}{\sqrt{N}} \qquad \text{(Eq. 2.1)}$$

Where $\bar{X}$ is the observed sample mean.

Z_p is the normal deviate, i.e. Z value corresponding to the desired confidence level (to be calculated from Appendix 1).

N = sample size

σ = population standard deviation.

It is apparent from the Eq. 2.1 that as N increases the width of the range decreases but as P increases the range becomes wider. High value of standard deviation also widens the range.

When the level of confidence desired is 95%, P is written as 0.95. In two-sided confidence interval, deviation can take place on both the sides, i.e. true mean can be more as well as less than the sample mean. For $P = 0.95$ or 95% confidence interval, if the confidence interval is two-sided, the values of Zp is taken as 97.5% area of the standard normal curve.

$$(1 + 0.95)/2 = 0.975$$

However, confidence interval changes depending on the sample chosen, although s.d. (σ) and N remain the same, $\bar{X}$ varies from sample to sample.

Confidence Interval with Unknown Standard Deviation

In Eq. 2.1, σ represented the true standard deviation. However, in most of the cases, true standard deviation is unknown and hence it is derived from sample data. In t distribution instead of σ, confidence interval of $\bar{X}$ depends on the sample standard deviation and the t value for a particular degree of freedom. Since the true standard deviation is not known, the chance of the sample mean coinciding with the true mean is not high. In other words, if a number of samples are taken from the same population, there is no guarantee that the standard deviation will be the same in every case. Hence, it is safer to represent the mean as a range or confidence interval for a particular probability value of t distribution.

$$P\% \text{ (confidence interval)} = \bar{X} \pm \frac{tS}{\sqrt{N}} \qquad \text{(Eq. 2.2)}$$

Here, t = value of t corresponding to the desired confidence level.
$\bar{X}$ is the observed sample mean
N is number of observation and S (s.d.) is sample standard deviation.

The values of t are obtained from cumulative t table (Appendix 2). For a particular degree of freedom, t table gives the value of t, under which a certain area of the curve occurs. The degree of freedom is usually taken as $N - 1$, where N is the sample size. As the value of N (number of observations in a sample) increases, the value of t (in the t table) decreases.

When true s.d. is known, the Z value is used in place of t value.

So the steps of assessing a confidence interval of mean for a population from a sample are:

Recording the sample size and estimation of sample mean.
↓
Choice of confidence level, i.e. 95% or 99% or 99.5%, etc.
↓
To ascertain whether true s.d. is known or unknown.
↓
Selection of the test.
↓
Getting the value of Z (for true s.d.)/t (for sample s.d.)
↓
Substituting the values in Eq. 2.1 or 2.2 (as is the case).
↓
Calculating the range along with proper unit.

HYPOTHESIS TESTING

What is Hypothesis Testing?

Statistical hypothesis testing is a useful method of assessing whether or not the observed difference in response between the groups (say placebo and treatment) could be attributed due to a genuine cause.

For example, when a new drug is tested for its efficacy, often it is compared against a placebo. Usually, patients or volunteers are taken with similar characteristics and divided randomly into groups. Then one group receives placebo while the other group receives the drug. The responses (e.g. change in blood sugar and blood pressure, etc.) are measured and the results of the two groups are compared to make a decision. However, often it is seen that some members of the placebo group show responses that are expected from the drug. Similarly, some members from the treatment group may not respond to the drug. These deviations from the expected result may be due to the bio-variation or error of measurement. If the difference between the effect of the treatment group and the placebo group is large, it apparently looks like that the drug has some effect. If the error (variation of response within the same group) is large then the possibility lies that the difference between the result of the treatment group and placebo group is also due to chance rather than any real cause. To come to a clear-cut conclusion about the efficacy of the drug from such overlapping result is difficult without statistical analysis. *Hypothesis testing is a statistical procedure that helps us in making a decision in such cases.*

What is the Rationale of Decision-Making?

When two products (e.g. drug and placebo) are different, it is expected that they would have different effects. However, the difference of effects may be intensified or reduced because of errors. By mistake, we may include a person in the drug group, who is resistant to the test drug and does not show any effect or we may choose a sensitive person in the placebo group, who just by thinking that he is under medication, may show some drug effect. Hence, instead of the quantitative difference, the ratio of the difference (of responses) of group means to that of error (within group variability) is taken as the basis for decision-making. The magnitude of the ratio is related to a probability statement. However, obtaining a real drug effect does not mean the drug has utility. A very small but real effect may not be sufficient to qualify a molecule as drug.

SOME IMPORTANT TERMS USED IN HYPOTHESIS TESTING

Null Hypothesis

Null hypothesis is a hypothetical statement about the sample parameters, which are evaluated by statistical methods. The sign H_0 is used to indicate it.

When we say H_0: $\mu_1 = \mu_2$, it indicates mean of the two treatments μ_1 and μ_2, (e.g. placebo and drug) are equal. In a comparison between drug and placebo, if null hypothesis is proved right, it indicates that the drug does not have any effect. If proved wrong, (i.e. rejected), the indication is that 'the result of the drug treatment group is different from that of placebo group'. So when null hypothesis is rejected, we say the difference is statistically significant. Like null hypothesis, there is an alternative hypothesis too. Alternative hypothesis is expressed by H_a. If null hypothesis is proved right, alternative hypothesis is proved wrong.

The expression for alternative hypothesis is: H_a: $\mu_1 \neq \mu_2$.

The α and β Error

In hypothesis testing the level of significance is to be specified. By convention when null hypothesis is rejected, we say there is a real difference between the groups but sometimes it may so happen that the groups compared are basically same and chance variations are erroneously interpreted as a significant or real difference. So there is always a small chance that the decision made on the basis of hypothesis testing is wrong. This error can happen for both decisions, acceptance as well as rejection. If the statistical test results in rejection of the null hypothesis, error that could be included in the decision is called α error.

The β error is associated with the probability of accepting the null hypothesis (H_0), i.e. declaring the result as similar, when they were actually different.

Level of Significance (P value)

This is the famous *P* value, widely cited in pharmaceutical literature. *P* value indicates the chances of being wrong in decision-making. The lesser the *P* value, greater is the correctness. Before starting a comparison, *P* value is to be specified. The lesser is the chosen *P* value, the greater is the reliability of the decision.

One-Tailed Test and Two-Tailed Test

One tail or two tails refer to the areas in the ends of distribution curves. Statistical distributions are symmetrical in nature and most of the values are near the mean. For example, take a batch of capsules. There will be some variation in the weight among individual capsules but deviation is not likely to be high. If the target weight of the batch is 250 mg and we examine 100 capsules from it, the chance is that most will have weight near 250 mg. There may be stray capsules, heavier and lighter than the target weight but the weight variation due to light weight capsules will be balanced by the heavy weight capsules and mean weight of the sample is likely to be near 250 mg, i.e. target mean. In other words, weight distribution pattern of the capsule will show mean and near mean values in the middle area of the curve and extreme values near the ends. Hence, the distribution curve of sample means has greater height in middle area of the curve and two tapering ends. The narrow tails/end part indicates that the probability of sample mean to fall in these end areas is rather slim. Suppose another company prepares the capsule of the same drug. If the products are similar, it is expected that the standard deviation and mean will be same in the new brand too. However, if the brands are different, the mean weight of the new brand can be either higher or lower than the mean weight of the old brand. In two-tailed test, we examine the possibility of this difference of means (weighted against the error of measurement) falling in either end of the normal curve. In one-tailed test, we have a preconceived notion that values in one brand are greater or lesser than other group and area of rejection lies at one end only.

The Critical Region

The concept of critical region is shown in Fig. 2.1. The critical region is usually taken as the symmetrical area in the tails of distribution with each tail containing $\alpha/2$ of the area for a two-tailed test. For one-tailed test it would be α% in the one tail area. The values of $\bar{X}$ that cause rejection of null hypothesis fall within this region and while stating a decision, we say significant at α% level, meaning that the probability of finding $\bar{X}$ (mean value of data set) in this area is α%.

Critical Region in Two-sided Test

If α is chosen as 5%, the critical region would be 2.5% area in both the tails of distribution for a two-sided test. In Z distribution, the cutoff point for this area is ± 1.96. For other distributions, if α chosen is 5%, the critical region would be

$$\pm 1.96 \times \frac{s.d.}{\sqrt{N}}$$

units away from mean value of the population. Suppose, the mean value obtained from a sample population is 5 and s.d. is 2.04. If the number of samples is 4, the critical region will constitute the values $\bar{X}$ that lie beyond the value of

$$5 \pm \frac{1.96 \times 2.04}{\sqrt{4}}.$$

Accordingly, the values of $\bar{X}$ below 3 and above 5 will cause rejection of null hypothesis. The shaded portion of the Fig. 2.1 shows the critical region where null hypothesis will be rejected for the test (95% confidence level). In a comparison, if the sample mean is found to be above 5 or below 3 the difference is too high to be of a similar batch and decision is, 'the two groups are significantly different'.

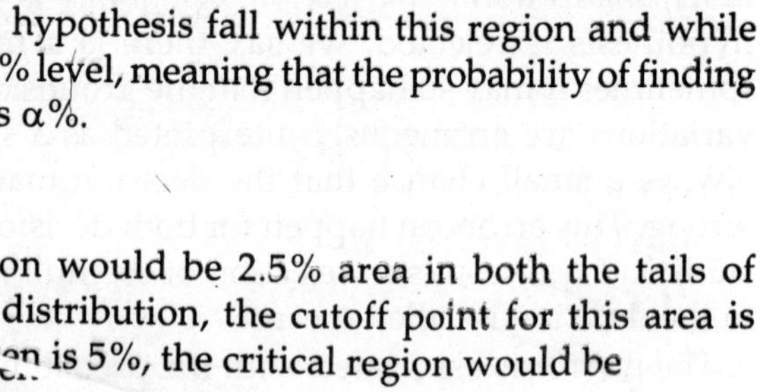

Fig. 2.1: Critical region of two-sided test (mean 5, s.d. 2.04, $N = 4$, $P < 0.05$)

Critical Region in a One-sided Test

For one-sided test with 95% confidence level, the entire area for rejection, (i.e. 5% area) for null hypothesis would lie at one end of the curve. However, this area can be at right side or at the left side. The Z value for cutoff point of 5% is

$$\text{either mean} + 1.65 \times \frac{s.d.}{\sqrt{N}} \text{ or mean} - 1.65 \times \frac{s.d.}{\sqrt{N}}.$$

How to Decide whether Test should be One-sided or Two-sided?

Statistical tests are usually two-sided. But in certain circumstances, one-sided tests are done. Suppose, we believe that the test batch of tablet is definitely of higher potency than the standard batch. There is no chance of its having lesser potency than the earlier batches. When we can justify such claims by logical reasoning, only one-sided test can be done. Here, the cutoff point for the critical region in the given example is

$$5 + \frac{1.65 \times 2.04}{\sqrt{4}} \text{ or } 6.68.$$

The t distribution looks like standard normal distribution curve but has more area in the tails. The distribution is more spread out and the shape depends on degree of freedom. As degree of freedom increases it resembles more and more like the standard normal distribution. When the degree of freedom is infinitely large, the t distribution takes the shape of standard normal distribution. Unlike the normal distribution, there is no transformation that converts all t distribution into one standard t distribution. The t table (Appendix 2) shows commonly used probability points of t distribution for various degrees of freedom.

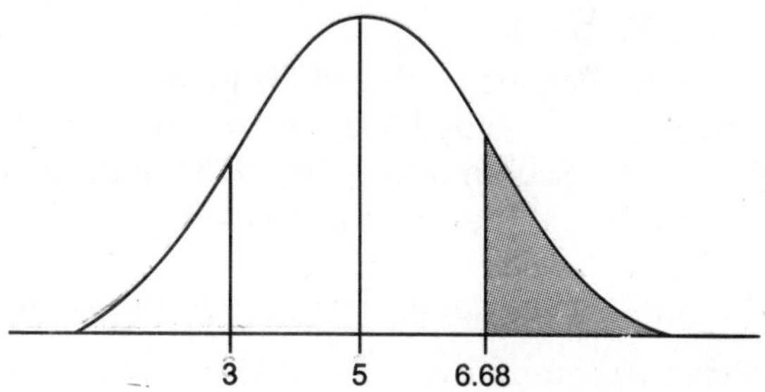

Fig. 2.2: Critical region of one-sided test (mean 5, s.d. 2.04, $N = 4$, $P < 0.05$)

Paired and Unpaired Tests

In designed experiments (e.g. test of efficacy of a drug molecule) treatments are given to different groups and results are compared. For this, individuals are randomly assigned into one or other groups. Each member of a group is a separate entity or independent of other members. They are not related or paired with any other experimental units. Such tests are called unpaired tests.

However, sometimes groups are formed in such a way that a member of one sample has a unique relationship with a particular member of the other sample or for both the groups, values are taken from the same experimental units. Blood pressure of the same person measured before and after drug treatment is an example. Such tests are called paired tests. Data recorded in such tests are the difference between the two observations.

Z Value and *t* Value

Z values and *t* values are obtained from *Z* and *t* tables respectively. When the standard deviation is known, we go for a *Z* test. If unknown and determined from the sample, we consult *t* table to ascertain the probability of an event.

Z table gives the area of the critical zone for a particular value of *Z*. The confidence or significance level of a statement is calculated from this cutoff area. So if we want a confidence level of 95%, we should look for the value that cuts off 5% of the area. In two-sided tests this would be the cutoff value for 2.5% area and for one-sided test 5% of area. *Z* table shows these values are ± 1.96 and ± 1.65 respectively. *Z* values and *t* values are obtained from *Z* and *t* tables respectively (Appendices 1 and 2).

The nature of *t* distribution is symmetrical with a mean of zero. However, exact values of *t* for a cutoff area (critical zone) depends upon the degree of freedom. For a two-sided test with degrees of freedom 8, the required *t* ratio for significance at 5% level is 2.31. It indicates that a vertical line drawn at the point 2.31 on the X-axis will cut off 2.5% area of the curve. This means for a two-tailed test with degrees of freedom 8, the calculated *t* ratio must be equal to or more than the value of 2.31 to be significant at the 5% level.

If the calculated value of *t* is greater than 2.31, the finding is significant at 5% level. Thus for a two-sided test, the experimental *t* value is to be compared with the *t* value given in the column-head of 0.975 but the column-head 0.95 should be selected for the comparison if the test is one-sided.

Common Comparisons Used in Pharmacy

Types of comparison or statistical test to be performed depend upon the objective of pharmaceutical experiment. There are different types of comparisons but commonly used types are discussed below.

1. Test of mean from a single population or comparison with a standard value.
2. Comparison between two independent groups (unpaired *t* tests).
3. Comparison between two related groups (paired *t* tests).
4. Comparison between more than two independent groups (ANOVA).

Test of mean from a single population or comparison with a standard value

This simple test can be divided into few steps.

Step 1: Objective of the experiment is to be defined and level of significance is to be chosen.

Step 2: Statement of the standard values with which comparison is to be done.

Step 3: *Standard deviation is known or to be estimated from the sample.* This step is crucial as the nature of standard deviation determines the type of test to be carried out.

Step 4: Determination of the sample statistic (mean and s.d.). Proper sampling is to be done, so that it represents the population being tested. Sample size or number of observation in the sample should be adequate to represent the population.

Step 5: If the standard deviation is known or given, *Z* ratio is calculated as per Eq. 2.3 and the value is compared with the values given in *Z* table for the specified level of significance.

$$Z = \frac{|\bar{X} - \mu_0|}{\sqrt{\frac{\sigma^2}{N}}} \qquad \text{(Eq. 2.3)}$$

In the above equation, numerator is the difference of sample and standard mean. The denominator is the standard deviation of the numerator.

The variance of $\bar{X}$ is equal to σ^2/N. Square root of variance is standard deviation.

The numerator is the difference of true mean and sample mean. As μ_0 (true mean) is constant, it should have no variance. Hence, Z ratio consists of a difference divided by standard deviation of mean. In most of the cases, the standard deviation is derived from historical data and treated as true process parameter. Suppose. production data of tablets over a period of 5 years show average weight and standard deviation is 50 and 2 mg respectively. These are considered as standard process parameters and hence regarded as known parameters. Sometimes, comparison is done with a hypothetical (e.g. label claim of a tablet or capsule) value too. However, when s.d. is not known, variance is estimated from sample data. In such cases, the sample variance is used (in the denominator) instead of the true variance and t test is performed as per Eq. 2.4.

$$t = \frac{|\bar{X} - \mu_0|}{\sqrt{\frac{S^2}{N}}} \qquad \text{(Eq. 2.4)}$$

Z ratio shows standard normal distribution which has a mean of 0 and variance of 1. The value of sample mean $\bar{X}$ that causes rejection of null hypothesis is given in Z table.

A worked out example for one sample test

Example 1: Given is the assay result for 10 randomly selected tablets (Table 2.1) obtained from a newly manufactured batch. If the mean and standard deviations obtained from historical data are 53 and 2.5 mg, is the current batch acceptable as same as the old batches?

Table 2.1: Assay result for 10 randomly selected tablets

Serial no.	*Tablet potency (mg)*
1	50.50
2	51.30
3	49.90
4	52.45
5	53.90
6	52.75
7	50.35
8	53.20
9	50.30
10	52.50
Mean	51.715
Variance	2.00
s.d.	1.415

As the s.d. is known, the test will be carried out according to Eq. 2.3.
The true s.d. (σ) is 2.5 mg, $\sigma^2 = 6.25$.

$$Z = \frac{|51.715 - 53|}{\sqrt{\frac{6.25}{10}}} = \frac{1.285}{0.790} = 1.625$$

For significance at 5% level, cutoff value for Z ratio is ± 1.96. Since the Z value calculated is 1.625 the values of the new batch appears to be same as the historical batches, the new batch is accepted to have similar potency as the old batches.

The cutoff point for the value of mean (significance at 5% level) in a two-sided Z test is

$$\mu \pm \frac{1.96 \times 2.5}{\sqrt{10}} = 53.0 \pm 1.54$$

The confidence interval is 51.46 to 54.54 mg. The sample mean (51.715 mg) is well within this range.

When the true s.d. is unknown, the test is carried out according to Eq. 2.4 using the s.d. obtained from the sample.

$$t = \frac{|51.715 - 53|}{\sqrt{\frac{2}{10}}} = \frac{1.285}{0.447} = 2.875$$

The value of t with a d.f. (10–1) is 2.26 (Appendix 2). Since, the t value calculated from the sample is 2.875 (greater than the cutoff value of 2.26), the potency of the new batch appears to be different from the historical batches.

The cutoff point for the value of mean (significance at 5% level) in a two-sided t test is

$$\mu \pm \frac{t \times S}{\sqrt{N}} \text{ or } 53 \pm \frac{2.26 \times 1.415}{\sqrt{10}}$$

So, the confidence interval is 53.0 ± 1.01 or 51.99 to 54.01. The value of sample mean (51.715 mg) falls outside this range.

Comparison of mean from two independent group test (unpaired test)

The assumption: The principal feature of this test is that the groups compared are independent in nature. In clinical and preclinical studies such tests are carried out, where both the groups have different members. It is assumed that within each group data are normally distributed. In other words, most of the sample units have value near the group mean and a few are away from that.

First, null hypothesis and α (error level) are set.

Secondly, a decision is taken about the type of test. If the variance of both groups is known, Z ratio is calculated as per Eq. 2.5.

$$Z = \frac{\overline{X}_1 - \overline{X}_2 - (\mu_1 - \mu_2)}{\sqrt{\sigma_1^2 / N_1 + \sigma_2^2 / N_2}} \qquad \text{(Eq. 2.5)}$$

Here, $\overline{X}_1$ and $\overline{X}_2$ are the sample means.
μ_1 and μ_2 are the true means of population 1 and population 2.
σ_1 and σ_2 are true standard deviations of population 1 and 2.
N_1 and N_2 are number of units in sample 1 and 2.
When $\mu_1 = \mu_2$ the equation reduces to

$$Z = \frac{|\overline{X}_1 - \overline{X}_2|}{\sqrt{\sigma_1^2 / N_1 + \sigma_2^2 / N_2}} \qquad \text{(Eq. 2.6)}$$

However, in two independent group tests, if the variances are unknown, they are calculated from sample data. To simplify the procedure, let us assume variance is same for each group. First, the variances are calculated and the two variances are pooled to get an estimate for common variance by using the following formula (Eq. 2.7).

$$S_p^2 = \frac{(N_1 - 1) S_1^2 + (N_2 - 1) S_2^2}{N_1 + N_2 - 2} \qquad \text{(Eq. 2.7)}$$

Here, S_p^2 is the common variance, estimated from sample data.
Finally, the t value is calculated by,

$$t = \frac{(X_1 - X_2) - (\mu_1 - \mu_2)}{\sqrt{S_p^2 / N_1 + S_p^2 / N_2}} \qquad \text{(Eq. 2.8)}$$

To ascertain the level of significance t table is to be referred. The degree of freedom is taken as $N_1 + N_2 - 2$. If the estimated t value is greater than the t value specified in the table (for a stated level of significance) the two populations are declared as different.

A worked out example of two independent group test

Example 2: Given below is the assay result (Table 2.2) obtained from two different capsule brands of a drug. Perform a test to decide whether they are similar with respect to potency.

Table 2.2: Assay results for capsules of brand *A* and brand *B*

Serial no.	*Brand A (mg)*	*Brand B (mg)*
1	65	62
2	79	75
3	76	77
4	80	72
5	82	69
6	85	72
Average	77.83	71.17
Sample variance	48.57	27.77
s.d	6.97	5.27

First, the pooled variance is calculated by using the Eq. 2.7

$$S_p^2 = \frac{6 \times 48.57 + 6 \times 27.77}{6+6-2} = 45.8$$

The t ratio is calculated by the Eq. 2.8

$$t = \frac{77.83 - 71.17}{\sqrt{\dfrac{45.8}{6} + \dfrac{45.8}{6}}} = \frac{6.66}{3.9} = 1.707$$

This t value is compared with the value obtained from t table with d.f. (6 + 6 – 2), i.e. 10.

In Appendix 2, the t value with d.f. 10 is 2.23 for a significance level of 5%.

As the t value obtained from the analysis is 1.70 (lesser than 2.23) the brands are not significantly different.

For the above test, we assumed that the variance is same for each group in addition to the usual assumptions of normality and independence of data. To assume equality of variances, a rule of thumb for moderate-sized samples (N ranging 10–20) is that the ratio of the two variances should not be greater than 3 to 4. However, if the two groups have different variances and variances are unknown (derived from sample as in Table 2.2) the t values needed for significance are different from those recorded in Appendix 2. In those cases, t value for significance is obtained from a special procedure known as Behrens-Fisher procedure. In this, the t value needed for significance is a weighted average of the appropriate t values with N_1 and N_2 degree of freedom.

Weighted average of t values is given by

$$t' = \frac{w_1 t_1 + w_2 t_2}{w_1 + w_2}$$

Here, w_1 and w_2 represent weights

$$w_1 = \frac{S_1^2}{N_1} \text{ and } w_2 = \frac{S_2^2}{N_2}$$

If number of samples in both the groups are same as in the current case, the critical value of t (value of t needed for significance) can be taken from t table (Appendix 2) but instead of d.f. 2 (N – 1), (i.e. 10) the value of d.f. should be taken as (N – 1) or 5.

At 5% level, this value of t is (d.f. 5) 2.57.

The t ratio calculated should have individual variance instead of pooled variance.

For the data of Table 2.2 (if the variances are considered unequal) the t value would be,

$$t = \frac{77.83 - 71.17}{\sqrt{\dfrac{48.57}{6} + \dfrac{27.77}{6}}} = \frac{6.66}{\sqrt{12.72}} = 1.87.$$

As the value calculated is lesser than 2.57, the decision is 'the brands are not different.'

Paired *t* Test

Paired *t* test is conducted for the comparison of means when the samples are related. Compared to unpaired test, paired *t* test is more sensitive as it can differentiate between much smaller differences. In paired *t* test, treatments are done in random order. Sometimes matching characteristics are chosen to have paired subjects. Often patients become their own control. For example, when an antihypertensive drug is tested for clinical efficacy, change in blood pressure after administration of medicine is recorded. The difference between pre- and post-treatment value is the data point and each patient is his own control. Similarly, results of bioavailability or bioequivalence study are best analyzed by paired *t* test.

The paired *t* test is the same as the one sample *t* test.

The formula for obtaining *t* is

$$t = \frac{\bar{\delta} - \Delta}{S/\sqrt{N}} \qquad \text{(Eq. 2.9)}$$

Here,

$\bar{\delta}$ = mean value of the observations (mean difference of pre- and post-treatment data.)

Δ = hypothetical difference

N = number of observations

S = standard deviation of observations

In clinical studies, a paired design indicates that each patient acts as his own control. Pairs can be devised in clinical trials by pairing patients with similar characteristics. Bioequivalence study where each subject is administered each test drug and a standard drug, is a paired design. The data points are obtained by taking the differences between the results for the two treatments on each subject. In estimation of drug effect too, initial reading is taken at the pretreatment level and another at the post-treatment. Here, some problem may arise as no single point can be assumed as control or a control group is lacking. The effect of time also influences experimental result. So randomization is extremely important for such studies to come up with a reliable decision.

A worked out example of paired t test

Paired *t* test is mostly used in bioavailability study; for example, to test a new formulation for bioavailability in comparison with a standard formulation. There may be biovariation among the subjects. So subjects are randomly divided into two groups. Each subject receives standard and test drug on two different occasions, the AUCs (area under the curve) are noted. The difference in AUC for two drugs (in the same subject) is recorded and analyzed by paired *t* test.

Example 3: Given below is the AUC of two drugs, tested in the same group of volunteers. Perform a test to decide whether the test formulation is better than the standard in terms of bioavailability.

Table 2.3: Results (AUC) of standard and test formulations

Subjects	*X (standard)*	*Y (test)*	*Difference of X and Y*	*X/Y*
1	120	140	20	0.86
2	130	150	20	0.86
3	160	193	33	0.83
4	154	184	30	0.84
5	126	134	08	0.94
6	174	197	23	0.88

So the average difference of X and Y (average of 4th column) = 22.33, s.d. = 8.82. In terms of ratio the average is 0.87, S = 0.039.

The null hypothesis is $H_0: \mu_1 - \mu_2 = 0$

$$t = \frac{22.83 - 0}{8.82/\sqrt{6}} = 6.20 \text{ (calculated as per Eq. 2.9)}$$

The calculated t value should be compared against the cutoff value of t for a degree of freedom $N - 1$. If the value obtained is higher than that value, the difference is significant. The cutoff point for t is 2.57 at 5% level. The value of t is much higher than that. So the test formulation is statistically different from the standard formulation.

Paired t test is also used for preclinical study. In some of the experiments, differences are important and in some others ratios of pre- and post-treatment data are more important. When datum used is X/Y ratio, the comparison is done against the hypothetical value of 1.

Example 4: Given below the results of two experimental formulations tested in the same group of animals. Calculate whether or not the formulations are bioequivalent?

Table 2.4: Results of a bioequivalence study

Code	*Formulation*		*Formulation*	
	(AUC) A	*(AUC) B*	*B-A*	*A/B*
1	126	164	38	0.77
2	158	182	24	0.87
3	160	191	31	0.84
4	102	103	1	0.99
5	200	196	−4	1.02
6	162	95	−67	1.71
Average			3.83	1.03
Standard deviation			38.46	0.34

$$t = \frac{\bar{\delta} - \Delta}{S/\sqrt{N}} \quad \text{(Eq. 2.9)}$$

$$t = \frac{1.03 - 1}{0.34/\sqrt{6}} = 0.22$$

Since the required t value for significance ($P < 0.05$) is (2.57), formulations are not statistically different.

Binomial Test or Chi-Square Test

Binomial experiments have only two possible outcomes, e.g. success or failure, right or wrong, liking or disliking. For comparing organoleptic properties like taste, smell, etc. such comparison is used. For example, if two products *A* and *B* are given to people for selecting the better one in a blinded test (judges won't know the name of the brand), some will prefer formulation *A* and others *B*. Decision is made by first finding proportion of the preferred products and finally comparing them with the expected proportion.

If the comparison is between two products, the null hypothesis H_0 assumes both products are equally preferred.

H_0: $P_a = P_b = 0.5$ (preference for *A* is equal to the preference for *B*)

Here the alternative hypothesis is: H_a: $P_a \neq 0.5$.

Say out of 30 people, 20 preferred *A* and 10 preferred *B*. The proportion of *A*'s success is 20/30 and *B*'s success is 10/30. Clearly there is a preference for *A* but whether this preference is statistically significant or not can only be decided by a statistical analysis. For this, the Z ratio is calculated from the following equation.

$$Z = \frac{|\hat{p} - p_0| - \dfrac{1}{2N}}{\sqrt{p_0 q_0 / N}} \qquad \text{(Eq. 2.10)}$$

Where,

$\hat{p}$ = observed proportion.

p_0 = expected or hypothetical proportion under the null hypothesis.

To calculate the probabilities for test of significance, table for standard normal distribution (Appendix 1) is used.

Chi-square tests are also used to compare proportions and counts. It is advantageous for two reasons:

1. Computations are easy.
2. Continuing corrections can be easily applied. It can be applied for comparing two independent groups.

A worked out example of chi-square test

Example 5: Formulation F1 and F2 are being compared. Both the formulations are given to two groups of people. Group *A* has 20 and group *B* has 30 members. Table 2.5 and 2.6 show the results of assessment. Do the groups have different preference?

In the group *A*, the formulation *F*1 is preferred by 16 people and in *B* the number is 12. A table is constructed first.

Table 2.5: Preference for formulation *F*1

	Group A	*Group B*	*Total*
Preference	16	12	28
Dislike	4	18	22
Total	20	30	50

Table 2.6: Preference for formulation *F*2

	Group A	*Group B*	*Total*
Preference	4	18	22
Dislike	16	12	28
Total	20	30	50

Though there are two tables, yet any one is sufficient for the calculation.

Based on the average, the expected preference can be calculated for each formulation.

Here, the expected number is the number if both the formulations have same proportion of preferences. Out of 50, total preference for *F*1 is 28.

So, in group *A* out of 20, expected preference for *F*1 is

$$\frac{28 \times 20}{50} = 11.2$$

Similarly, the expected preference for *F*1 in group *B* is

$$\frac{28 \times 30}{50} = 16.8$$

Groups	*A*	*B*	*Total*
Expected number of preferences for *F*1	11.2	16.8	28
Expected number of disliking for *F*1	8.8	13.2	22

Another table needs to be constructed with the expected values of formulation *F*2.

In group *A* out of 20, expected preference for *F*2 is

$$\frac{22 \times 20}{50} = 8.8.$$

In group *B* out of 30, expected preference for *F*2 is

$$\frac{22 \times 30}{50} = 13.2.$$

The χ^2 can be computed as

$$\Sigma \frac{(O - E)^2}{E}.$$

Or
$$\chi^2 = (O - E)^2 \left(\frac{1}{E_1} + \frac{1}{E_2} + \frac{1}{E_3} + \frac{1}{E_4} \right) \quad \text{(Eq. 2.11)}$$

Where, O and E represent the observed and expected value of a formulation in a cell (particular group). E_1, E_2, E_3, E_4 represent expected values in each cell. There are two formulations tested in groups. So there are four cells in this example. So the value of χ^2 is

$$\frac{(16-11.2)^2}{11.2} + \frac{(12-16.8)^2}{16.8} + \frac{(4-8.8)^2}{8.8} + \frac{(18-13.2)^2}{13.2}.$$

The numerator in each term is same, i.e. $(4.8)^2$. So can be simplified as:

$$\chi^2 = (4.8)^2 = \left(\frac{1}{11.2} + \frac{1}{16.8} + \frac{1}{8.8} + \frac{1}{13.2} \right) = 7.7922.$$

In general, the degrees of freedom for an $R \times C$ contingency table is $(R-1) \times (C-1)$ where R and C are the rows and columns in the table.

Appendix 5 gives the values of chi-square for particular degrees of freedom at different probability levels. Since number of rows and columns are both 2 in the current problem, the degree of freedom is $(2-1)(2-1) = 1$. To be significant at 5% level the required χ^2 value is 3.84. Hence, the decision is 'two groups have different preferences'.

ANALYSIS OF VARIANCE (ANOVA)

ANOVA is a general method of analyzing data from designed experiments, where two or more group means are compared. The t test is a special case of ANOVA, where only 2 group means are compared. In a clinical study, the t test is usually done, when two treatments are randomly assigned to different experimental units. However, when number of groups exceeds two, ANOVA is performed.

Statistical analysis depends on designs. So certain analysis is relevant for certain designs.

In Pharmacy, one-way ANOVA is used when it is desired to find out the equality of treatment means.

Groups are formed by randomly assigning subjects in one or other groups. Then treatments are done, each group receiving different treatment. The null hypothesis assumes that the effects in the groups are same and is written as H_0: $\mu_1 = \mu_2 = \mu_3$.

ANOVA separates the total variability in a set of data into component parts.

Though desirable, having equal number of subjects is not necessary in this design.

One-Way ANOVA

One-way ANOVA is represented by the model

$$Y_{ij} = \mu + G_i + \varepsilon_{ij} \quad \text{(Eq. 2.12)}$$

Y_{ij} = any specific response of an experiment. The index ij indicates jth response in treatment group i. Hence, Y_{23} means third response in second treatment group.

μ = overall mean

G_i = deviation of the *i*th group mean from the overall mean.

ε_{ij} = random error in the experiment.

Suppose, a particular drug is being tested in three groups.

As the drug administered is same to all three groups they should produce identical responses. But the response found was different in different individuals because subjects even if matched for similar characteristics, have biovariation, and there may be errors in measurement too.

Hence, variation in response does not mean treatments are different. Even if the responses are different, a properly done ANOVA should show that there is no difference.

ANOVA analyses the variances in data and divide it in two sections.

1. Variance due to error
2. Variance due to intrinsic property of treatments.

The second type of variance, if large gives testimony that the groups are different in nature.

Example 6: Three groups each having two subjects are treated with 3 formulations of the same drug. The intensity of the drug effects is graded numerically, (i.e. no effect is 0 and greater effects are indicated with higher numbers) in Table 2.7. Are the formulations statistically similar with respect to drug effect?

Table 2.7: Effect of drug in different groups

Group 1 (n = 2) effect	*Group 2 (n = 2) effect*	*Group 3 (n = 2) effect*
0	2	10
2	4	12
Mean = 1	Mean = 3	Mean = 11

We can determine the grand average (μ) by averaging all the values

$$(0 + 2 + 4 + 2 + 10 + 12) = 30/6 = 5.$$

The same can be determined by averaging the group means too.

$$1 + 3 + 11 = 15/3 = 5$$

Group means have symbol Y_i.

Analysis is divided into the following steps.

Determination of Total Sum of Squares (TSS)

The difference of the first value 0 from mean is (5 – 0) = 5. When it is squared, the value becomes 25, which is much higher than the simple difference. Similarly, difference of all values from the grand mean is calculated, squared and added to obtain *total sum of squares* (TSS).

Deviations, both positive and negative types, may happen due to errors. So must be represented in the calculation of total variances.

Squaring of the values has two advantages.

1. All values become positive. There is no chance of a negative deviation canceling the positive deviations.
2. By squaring a small deviation becomes insignificant and a large deviation gets magnified.

The value 0.1 squared is 0.01, which is much lesser than 0.1, but if the deviation is 2 then squaring makes it 4, a greater value.

According to the ANOVA model,

$$\Sigma (Y_{ij} - \bar{Y})^2 = \Sigma (Y_{ij} - \bar{Y}_i)^2 + \Sigma N_i (\bar{Y}_i - \bar{Y})^2 \qquad \text{(Eq. 2.13)}$$

The term on the left hand side shows the total sum of squares, written as $\Sigma (Y_{ij} - \bar{Y})^2$.

$$\text{TSS} = (0-5)^2 + (2-5)^2 + (2-5)^2 + (4-5)^2 + (10-5)^2 + (12-5)^2 = 118$$

On the right hand side there are two terms. The first term represents the total difference of the individual values from the respective group means squared. This is called within sum of squares.

Mean for group 1 is 1. So, within sum of square for group 1 is

$$(0-1)^2 + (2-1)^2 = 1 + 1 = 2$$

Similarly, mean for group 2 is 3, hence the value is

$$(3-2)^2 + (3-4)^2 = 1 + 1 = 2$$

Mean for 3rd group is 11, so,

$$(10-11)^2 + (12-11)^2 = 1 + 1 = 2$$

So the value of the 1st term (within sum of square of all groups added) is

$$2 + 2 + 2 = 6$$

In the second part N_i (number of observations per group) is 2 for each group, as there are 2 subjects in each group. The grand mean is 5. So the total sum of squares is

$$= 2\,[(1-5)^2 + (3-5)^2 + (11-5)^2]$$

$$= 2\,(16 + 4 + 36) = 112.$$

TSS can be obtained by adding

$$\Sigma (Y_{ij} - \bar{Y}_i)^2 \text{ and } \Sigma N_i (Y_i - \bar{Y})^2$$

$$6 + 112 = 118.$$

The total sum of squares (TSS) was divided into two parts. Within treatment sum of squares (WSS) is taken as errors. The logic is that within the same group the treatment is same. So here all values should be same and any deviation or variation in results is positively due to errors. Within treatment sum of squares divided by the appropriate degree of freedom is the pooled variance.

The ratio of between treatment mean square (BSS) to within treatment mean square (WSS) is a measure of treatment differences.

The short cut formula for calculation of TSS is

$$\Sigma Y^2 - \frac{(\Sigma Y)^2}{N}. \quad \text{(Eq. 2.14)}$$

$\frac{(\Sigma Y)^2}{N}$ is the grand total of all observations squared, divided by total number of observations. This is known as the correction term (CT).

The between treatment sum of squares (BSS) is calculated as

$$\Sigma \frac{T_i^2}{N_i} - CT. \quad \text{(Eq. 2.15)}$$

T_i is the sum of observations in treatment group 'i' and N_i is the number of observations in the treatment group 'i'.

As total sum of square is the sum of within treatment sum of squares (WSS) and between treatment sum of squares (BSS), the within treatment sum of squares (WSS) can be calculated as the difference between TSS and BSS.

$$\text{WSS} = \text{TSS} - \text{BSS}$$

ANOVA table gives the source, degrees of freedom (d.f.), sum of squares (SS), mean square (MS) and the probability based on the statistical test of F ratio. Note that the more is the degrees of freedom, the less is the chance of error.

For the given example the table would look like,

Table 2.8: ANOVA table for Example 6

Source	*Degree of freedom*	*SS*	*MS*	*F*
Between groups	2	118	56	28*
Within groups	3	6	2	

*$P < 0.05$

In this case, there are total 3 groups. So degree of freedom for between groups (BSS) is 3 – 1 = 2. In each of the groups there are 2 observations. So the d.f. in within group sum of squares is (number of total observations – number of groups) = (6 – 3) = 3. The distribution of BMS/WMS ratio is called the F distribution. Hence F value obtained is 56/2 = 28. The required F value for significance is (F table for upper 5% value) is 9.55. Hence formulations are not statistically same.

The assumptions underlying the statistical test ANOVA are independence of errors, equality of variance and normally distributed errors.

When the treatments are identical, the term due to treatment differences should be zero and BSS should be approximately equal to WSS. However, random errors make the terms unequal even if treatments are identical. F distribution is an asymmetric distribution with long tails at large values of F.

The upper 5% significance tables are used for one-sided test.

Post-Tests of ANOVA

Once the one-way ANOVA shows a significant F value, usually post-tests are carried out.

A significant F ratio only indicates that the groups are not similar. But it does not indicate whether all groups are dissimilar or some are similar to one to another but different from other. For this, tests have to be carried out, where two groups are compared at a time.

Suppose, we like to compare the methods B and C with A (standard method). The mean results of A, B and C are μ_1, μ_2 and μ_3 respectively.

The null hypothesis will be

$$H_0 = \mu_1 = \mu_2 = \mu_3$$

For this, the usual t test procedure is followed as in comparison of two groups. However, the estimate of variance should come from all the groups and not only from the two groups, which are compared to each other.

The pooled within mean square term of ANOVA should be taken as estimate of variance. If three methods are to be compared, confusion may arise from three different t tests.

We may have results indicating,

A is not same as B, i.e. $A > B$ or $A < B$.

A is same as C, i.e. $A = C$.

B is same as C, i.e. $B = C$.

As both A and B are equal to C, A should be equal to B. But t tests, in which the standard deviations are obtained from the data of comparing groups only, may show this type error, i.e. ($A > B$ or $A < B$).

The confusion can only be solved if all three groups are brought to a common platform. The pooled within mean square term of ANOVA represents the common error in all groups and should be used for comparison in place of standard deviation. There are a number of post-tests for comparing the groups, e.g. Dunnett's test, Bonferroni's tests, etc.

Two-Way Anova

Two-way ANOVA is an extension of the paired t test but it is used where more than two treatment groups are to be compared. It is extensively used in clinical trials, where each patient evaluates two or more types of treatment.

This treatment takes into consideration the difference between the patients. In one-way ANOVA, we assume all the subjects receiving drug are similar but in reality same dose of the same drug may elicit different response to different people. Two-way ANOVA can detect the variation in the recipient as well as variation in the treatment.

Example 7: Given below is an example where results are tabulated for three formulations *DF* – 1, *DF* – 2 and *DF* – 3, tested by 5 methods. Perform two-way ANOVA to detect the difference in methods as well as the difference in formulations.

Table 2.9: Results of analysis of three dosage forms using 5 methods

Method	*(DF – 1)* Y_1	*(DF – 2)* Y_2	*(DF – 3)* Y_3	*Row-total*	*Row sq*	Y_1 *squared*	Y_2 *squared*	Y_3 *squared*
1st	16	18	20	54	2916	256	324	400
2nd	13	15	16	44	1936	169	225	256
3rd	15	17	16	48	2304	225	289	256
4th	10	12	13	35	1225	100	144	169
5th	18	17	19	54	2916	324	289	361
Total	72	79	84	235	11297	1074	1271	1442
Total sq	5184	6241	7056	18481				

Total sum of squares is obtained by summing the squares of individual values, and subtracting the correction term from it.

$$TSS = \Sigma X^2 - CT$$

In columns 6, 7 and 8 individual values are squared. All these column-totals are added to find the value of ΣX^2.

In this example, the value is 3787.

Correction term is sum of all values squared (ΣX^2) divided by the total number of observations *N*.

Sum of all values is 235. Number of observation is 15.

So the correction term = $(235)^2/15 = 55225/15 = 3681.665$.

Total sum of square (TSS) = 3787 – 3681.665 = 105.3333.

Between method sum of squares is obtained from CSS, i.e. sum of the squared values of column-total Y_1, Y_2 and Y_3 divided by number of rows and subtracting the correction term from it.

$$\text{Column sum of squares (CSS)} = \frac{\Sigma C_j^2}{R} - CT$$

Column totals are 72, 79 and 84 and number of rows is 5.

So, $[(72)^2 + (79)^2 + (84)^2]/5 - 3681.665$.

$$18481/5 - 3681.665$$

$$3696.2 - 3681.665 = 14.53$$

Similarly, between formulation sum of squares can be obtained by RSS, i.e. summing square of rows total, dividing it with number of columns and subtracting the correction term from it.

$$RSS = \frac{R_i^2}{C} - CT$$

Sum of rows squared = 11297.

Rows of sum of square = (11297)/3 – 3681.665

= 3765.667 – 3681.665 = 84

So residual sum of square = total sum of squares – column sum of square – rows sum of square.

105.33 – 84 – 14.53 = 6.8

Table 2.10: ANOVA table of Example 7

Source	*Degree of freedom*	*Sum of squares*	*Mean sum of squares*	F^a
Between formulation	2	14.53	7.26	8.44
Between methods	4	84	21	24.41
Residual	8 (C × R)*	6.8	0.86	

* The degree of freedom of residual sum of squares is ($C \times R$) where C = number of columns, R = number of rows.

To look for the value of $F^{2/8}$ we have to consult Appendix 3 for significance at 5% level and Appendix 4 for 1% level. For $F^{2/8}$, we have to look for the value under the column-head 2 in the row number 8.

From the F table, we can see $F^{2/8}$ at 5% level has value of 4.46 and 8.65 at 1% level.

So formulations are different from each other at 5% level.

For $F^{4/8}$, the values needed for significance are 3.84 and 7.01 at 5% and 1% level. As the F ratio obtained is 24.41, it can be said that the methods are significantly different from each other at 1% level.

BIBLIOGRAPHY

1. Daniel W Wayne: *Biostatistics: A Foundation for Analysis in Health Sciences*, Seventh edition, John Wiley and Sons, 1999.
2. De, Muth James E, Basic statistics and pharmaceutical statistical applications, Marcel Dekker, Inc, 1999.
3. Gurumani N: *An Introduction to Biostatistics*, Second edition, 2005.
4. Sanford Bolton, *Practical and Clinical Applications*, Third edition, Marcel Dekker, Inc, 1997.

3 Linear Regression and Correlation

INTRODUCTION

Application of regression and correlation is quite common in pharmacy. But often students use these two terms interchangeably. Though the terms are related, there is a subtle difference between the two concepts. This chapter tries to analyze the similarities, differences as well as applications of these concepts in pharmacy.

CONCEPT OF REGRESSION ANALYSIS

What is Linear Regression Analysis?

Linear regression analysis investigates the relationship between two variables X and Y, where one variable Y is known to depend on the value of the other variable X. The best-known example of regression analysis in pharmacy is the making of standard curve for a drug by the method of UV absorption. We know that in drugs with chromophores, the quantity of the absorbed light depends upon the concentration of drug solution. Here light absorption is the effect, which depends on the concentration of the drug (cause). However, application of this functional relationship is based on a prior knowledge that the variables are linearly related. Linear regression analysis just ascertains the quantitative dependence of the response variable (dependent variable) on the independent variable.

Regression analysis assumes that a relationship exists and investigates the quantitative aspect of that relationship. It assesses the parameters that describe the relationship, i.e. the value of slope and intercept.

Application of Linear Regression in Pharmacy

To describe the relationship between variables (where the functional relationship is known to be linear).

To represent or predict a trend where the extent of response is unknown, e.g. the possible pharmacological response of the drug at a future time.

For prediction of stability.

To describe dose-response relationship.

For fitting of pharmacokinetic data (linear regression).

Rationale of Linear Regression Analysis

A straight line is described by the equation:

$$Y = A + BX$$

Here A is the intercept (the value of Y when $X = 0$), B is the slope ($\Delta Y/\Delta X$), and X and Y are independent and dependent variables. As B indicates the slope of the line and A the intercept, when both A and B are specified, the straight line is specified. But in real experiments assessment of these two parameters without error is not easy. Data obtained from real experiments contain errors and all the experimental points may not fall on the same straight line. A line drawn by eye on the basis of individual perception may be erroneous. In N point observation, we have N pairs of X, Y. When the values of Y, for different values of X, do not fall on the same straight line, drawing a single line becomes difficult. Hence the best-fit line is chosen on the basis of statistics, which is known as regression analysis.

Since Y is known to depend on X in a linear relationship, all the values of Y for the corresponding values of X should fall on the same line. But they deviate due to error and errors can be positive as well as negative.

Example 1: Let's assume for simplicity's sake, a relationship where $Y = 3X$ (intercept is 0). This means if X has values of 1, 2 or 3, the true values of Y are 3, 6 and 9 respectively. However, due to experimental error, the values recorded are different.

Table 3.1: The true and experimental value of *Y* for *X*

Value of X	*True value of Y*	*Experimental values of Y*
1	3	2
2	6	6
3	9	9

Note that in real life we do not have the true values and the relationship or the extent of Y's dependence on X is often ascertained by experimental values only. Table 3.1 shows the experimental values of Y to be 2, 6 and 9. In this case, we can have three lines.

1. A line passing 2 and 6. Here the slope $B = 4$, the point 9 is ignored.
2. A line passing through 6 and 9 ($B = 3$), the point 2 is ignored.
3. A line passing through 2 and 9 ($B = 3.5$), the point 6 is ignored.

Since each line accommodates 2 data points, it is impossible to choose one in favor of the other two. As every point has been generated by the same experiment it is logical that each should get equal importance. Linear regression analysis saves us from this dilemma. By analysis of data, it creates a regression line from which sum of squares of linear distances of each point is the least. This best-fit line is drawn in such a way that all the points are close to the line, if not on it.

However, if the experimental values are far from the true values (experimental error is large), the generated line is bound to be erroneous. Yet regression analysis will help us in taking a decision.

While calculating for the best-fit line, the deviations on the negative side and deviations on the positive side are given equal weightage. Squaring makes all the values positive. A smaller difference is minimized and a higher difference is magnified by squaring. Hence, for calculation of variance in data, squares of the vertical distances are taken into consideration. A regression line is the best-fit line from which sum of the squares of the vertical distances of each point is minimum. The sum of squares is expressed as $\Sigma (y - Y)^2$ where y denotes the experimental values of dependent variable and Y, the corresponding values on best-fit line.

Assumption of Linear Regression

1. A linear relationship exists between X (independent variable) and Y (dependent variable) and the relationship is described by the equation,

$$Y = A + BX \qquad \text{(Eq. 3.1)}$$

2. The independent variable is measured accurately. Hence, it is considered error-free.
3. The observed values of Y are normally distributed around the mean.
   Since Y is a function of X, ideally for particular value of X, Y should have a specific value. But as we measure Y several times, there can be some variation in it. Some values of Y can be higher than real value while others can be lower. If a specific value of Y is measured a number of times we will be getting a cluster of values where most of the values will be close to the real value, (i.e. within a close range) and a few may be very high or very low. In statistical term the observed values of Y are normally distributed around the mean, i.e. the true value of Y.
4. In real experiments, values obtained for Y for each value of X rarely match the true value of Y. Regression analysis assumes the extent of variation of Y against each value of X is constant.

Calculation of Best-fit Line

Throughout the chapter four letters X, Y, A, B are extensively used. To clarify any confusion regarding the use of these letters the meanings are given below.

X = independent variable.
$\bar{X}$ = mean value of X.
y = experimentally determined value of dependent variable Y.
Y = corresponding values of y on the best-fit line.
a = sample estimate of true intercept.
A = mean value of a.
b = sample estimate of true slope.
B = mean value of b.

Applying the method of calculus, the slope and intercept of the best-fit line can be determined. According to this, when y represents the actual experimental points and Y represents the corresponding points on the fitted line, and the slope of the fitted line is given by:

$$b = \frac{\Sigma(X - \bar{X})(y - \bar{y})}{\Sigma(X - \bar{X})^2} \qquad \text{(Eq. 3.2)}$$

$\bar{X}$ = mean *X*.

$\bar{y}$ = mean *Y*.

X and *y* are individual data points.

However, regression line considers each and every data pair. Given *N* pair of *X* and *y*, the best-fit line can be defined as the line, which minimizes the sum of squares of the vertical distances of each point from the fitted line.

Let us assume, on the best-fit line, the value of *y* is 5 at X = 2. If the observed value of *y* is 3 at X = 2, vertical distance between the real and observed point will be 3 – 5 = –2. Squaring this will make the value 4.

In the above example (Table 3.1), if X has values 1, 2 and 3, the average or $\bar{X}$ will be 2.

The slope by definition is $\Delta Y/\Delta X$.

$$\frac{(y - \bar{y})}{(X - \bar{X})}$$

If the numerator and denominator are multiplied by same value the ratio remains same.

So both are multiplied by $(X - \bar{X})$.

So, slope (*b*) is the averaged ratio of all these points.

$$b = \frac{\Sigma(X - \bar{X})(y - \bar{y})}{\Sigma(X - \bar{X})^2} \quad \text{as given in Eq. 3.2}$$

b is the slope of best-fit line. If the relation is $Y = bX$, the true value of *Y* corresponding to $\bar{X}$ is $b\bar{X}$.

Hence intercept,

$$a = \bar{y} - b\bar{X} \qquad \text{(Eq. 3.3)}$$

There is a shortcut computing formula too, in which the slope is calculated as:

$$b = \frac{N\Sigma Xy - (\Sigma X)(\Sigma y)}{N\Sigma X^2 - (\Sigma X)^2} \qquad \text{(Eq. 3.4)}$$

Here *N* is the number of *X*, *y* pairs.

The best-fit line is described as $Y = a + bX$ where the values of *a* and *b* are determined from Eqs 3.3 and 3.4.

Error of Best-fit or Least Square Line

For obtaining a standard curve where the relationships between X and *y* are linear, Eq. 3.2 is adequate.

But in pharmaceutical research, sometimes there are situations where the relationship is not linear like plasma concentration versus time profile or drug-response assays. Experimental results deviate from linearity because of two reasons:

1. The true nature of relationship is not linear.
2. Error of measurement

In those cases, we need to investigate whether or not two variables (independent and dependent) are linearly related. This is done by correlation studies. Moreover, when linear relationship is established, sometimes we get intercept, which may be due to errors.

While drawing a line, we have two options:

1. We can make the line to pass through zero.
2. Allow the line to have an intercept *A*.

But which option is better remains unanswered until the statistical test for slope and intercept is performed. To perform these tests, we need to have estimates of variance for intercept and slope.

Determination of the Variances of Intercept and Slope

There is always a possibility that the *X*, *y* pairs obtained from the experiments contain errors. So, both intercept and slope may have errors, as they were determined from experimental values. Whether the intercept has been obtained due to error or a true reason can be determined by analysis of variance.

As per the assumption of linear regression, sample estimates of slope (*b*) and intercept (*a*) are normally distributed with means equal to *B* and *A*.

The true variance of *A* is denoted by σ_a^2 and that of *B* by σ_b^2.

Using the method of calculus, the variance of *A* (intercept) is derived as:

$$\sigma_a^2 = \sigma_{Y,x}^2 \left[\frac{1}{N} + \frac{\bar{X}^2}{\Sigma\left(X - \bar{X}\right)^2} \right] \qquad \text{(Eq. 3.5)}$$

$$\sigma_b^2 = \frac{\sigma_{Y,x}^2}{\Sigma\left(X - \bar{X}\right)^2} \qquad \text{(Eq. 3.6)}$$

In Eqs 3.5 and 3.6,

σ_a^2 = variance estimate of *A* (intercept).

σ_b^2 = variance estimate of *B* (slope).

$\sigma_{Y,x}^2$ = variance of the response variable *Y*.

Note that, the left side of the Eq. 3.5 represents the variance of *A*, whereas $\sigma_{Y,x}^2$, at the right side is the variance of dependent variable, i.e. *Y*. Equations 3.5 and 3.6 clearly indicate that the variance of intercept (*a*) and slope (*b*) both depends on the variability of *Y*. When $\sigma_{Y,x}^2$ is unknown, the variances of *a* and *b* can be estimated by substituting

$$S_{Y,x}^2 \text{ for } \sigma_{Y,x}^2.$$

$\sigma_{Y,x}^2$ is the variance of *y* estimated from the sample *X*, *y* pairs.

If the values of *Y* vary widely, the experimental points are far from the points on the least square line and the estimated variance is high. If the experimental points are close to least square line, the estimated variability is minimal. When the points exactly match the points of best-fit line, estimated variance of Y becomes zero. An unbiased estimate of $\sigma^2_{Y,x}$ is obtained from the sum of squares of the deviations of the observed values (y) from that of the fitted lines.

The variance of Y can be determined from the sample by summing the squared deviations of y (observed values of Y) from the corresponding value of Y on the best-fit line and dividing it by the degree of freedom (Eq. 3.7).

$$S^2_{Y,x} = \frac{\Sigma (y - Y)^2}{N - 2} = \frac{\Sigma (y - \bar{y})^2 - b^2 \left[\Sigma (X - \bar{X})^2\right]}{N - 2} \qquad \text{(Eq. 3.7)}$$

Here y and Y represent the observed and predicted values of the dependent variable (Y) on the least square line respectively. The variance of y ($S^2_{Y,x}$) has $N - 2$ degrees of freedom because two parameters are estimated from the data.

To understand Eq. 3.7, we have to remember that the best-fit line has the equation ($Y = a + bX$). So, for X_i, the ith value of X, the value Y on the least square line should be $bX_i + a$.

Similarly, the value of Y for $\bar{X}$ (the mean value of $\bar{X}$) is $b\bar{X} + a$.

So, the difference of y (experimental value of Y) from $\bar{Y}$ (the mean value of Y) on the least square line is $b\bar{X} - bX_i$.

By squaring we get $b^2 (\bar{X} - X_i)^2$, which represents the squared distance of a specific value of Y from that of mean value of Y.

So, the sum of squared deviations is $b^2 \Sigma (X - \bar{X})^2$.

Similarly, the sum of the squared deviations of the observed values of y from that of $\bar{y}$ is given by $\Sigma (y - \bar{y})^2$.

Hence, the unbiased sample estimate of variance $S^2_{Y,x}$ is obtained from the sum of squares of deviations of the observed points from the fitted line with the equation.

$$\frac{\Sigma (y - \bar{y})^2 - b^2 \left[\Sigma (X - \bar{X})^2\right]}{N - 2}$$

When the real variance is unknown, $S^2_{Y,x}$ is substituted in Eq. 3.5 in place of $\sigma^2_{Y,x}$ to obtain S^2_a.

$$S^2_a = S^2_{Y,x} \left[\frac{1}{N} + \frac{\bar{X}^2}{\Sigma (X - \bar{X})^2}\right] \qquad \text{(Eq. 3.8)}$$

Similarly, the sample estimate of variance of slope (S^2_b) is obtained from the sum of squares of deviation of the observed points from the fitted line too.

$$S^2_b = \frac{S^2_{Y,x}}{\Sigma (X - \bar{X})^2} \qquad \text{(Eq. 3.9)}$$

Test of Intercept

The variance of intercept and slope determined by Eqs 3.8 and 3.9 are used for the test of slope and intercepts. To know whether the intercept is by error or really due to a reason the t test is performed. Null hypothesis assumes that intercept (A) is zero, which is written H_0: $A = 0$, whereas the alternative hypothesis is H_0: $A \neq 0$.

If null hypothesis is rejected, the intercept is real. This is two-sided test. If A is not zero, it can be lesser (cuts Y-axis at negative value) or greater (cuts Y-axis at positive value) than zero.

A t test is carried out to decide the point.

$$t_{df} = \frac{|a - \alpha|}{\sqrt{S_a^2}} \qquad \text{(Eq. 3.10)}$$

a = actual intercept

α = hypothetical intercept, i.e 0.

t_{df} = t statistic with df $N - 2$. N represents the number of X, y pairs.

S_a^2 = sample estimate of the variance of A as per Eq. 3.8.

For significance, the value of t obtained from Eq. 3.10 should be compared against the corresponding t value (Appendix 1).

Test of Slope

The test of slope for the least square line is of extreme importance in pharmacy. Often in dissolution studies, we use the value of slope to calculate the extent of drug release. Here, a slight mistake in value of slope may get multiplied many times. Hence, the magnitude of the slope is of special importance and needs to be determined accurately. Test of slope shows whether it is obtained by chance or due to a real cause. Sometimes, we want to be sure that the fitted line has a slope other than zero. At other times we may be interested in knowing whether the slope is other than 1. A slope of 1 indicates amount recovered (assay) is equal to the amount in the sample. If the null hypothesis assumes, the value of slope is 1, it is written as H_0: $B = 1$, alternative hypothesis is H_0: $B \neq 1$.

Similarly, in the test for slope (b),

$$t_{df} = \frac{|b - B|}{\sqrt{S_b^2}} \qquad \text{(Eq. 3.11)}$$

b = slope of the least-square line

B = hypothetical slope, i.e. 1.

t_{df} = t statistic with df $N - 2$. N represents the number of X, y pairs.

S_b^2 = sample estimate of the variance of B as per Eq. 3.9.

Like in the test for intercept the t value should be compared against corresponding t value in Appendix 1, for a stated level of significance.

Example 2: Perform the test for slope and intercept using the values of X and Y given in Table 3.2.

Table 3.2: Table for calculation of slope and intercept

Observations	X	*y*	X^2	Xy
1	1	6	1	6
2	2	7	4	14
3	3	10	9	30
4	4	13	16	52
5	5	16	25	80
Sum of the columns	15	52	55	182
Average	3.0	10.4		

Table 3.2 gives the values of observed X, y pairs. From this, slope and intercept are determined first then test for slope and intercept is performed.

$$\Sigma X = 15$$
$$\Sigma Y = 52$$
$$\bar{X} = 3$$
$$\bar{y} = 10.4$$
$$\Sigma Xy = 182$$
$$\Sigma X^2 = 55$$
$$N = 5$$
$$(X - \bar{X})^2 = 4 + 1 + 0 + 1 + 4 = 10$$

Similarly, $(y - \bar{y})^2 = 69.2$

$$t_{df} = \frac{|b - B|}{\sqrt{S_b^2}}$$

The formula for the slope is

$$b = \frac{N\Sigma Xy - (\Sigma X)(\Sigma y)}{N\Sigma X^2 - (\Sigma X)^2}$$

$$b = 2.6$$

Similarly, a is determined from Eq. 3.3.

$$a = \bar{y} - b\bar{X} \tag{Eq. 3.3}$$

$$a = 10.4 - 2.63 = 2.6$$

To know whether or not the slope is due to error, we have to perform the test for slope.

For this, variance of Y is to be determined from the sample data (Eq. 3.7).

$$S_{Y,x}^2 = \frac{\Sigma(y - Y)^2}{N - 2} = \frac{\Sigma(y - \bar{y})^2 - b^2\left[\Sigma(X - \bar{X})^2\right]}{N - 2}$$

$$= (69.2 - 2.62.610)/3$$

$$= 0.533$$

Next, using the variance from the sample data, we have to determine the variance of intercept (a) using Eq. 3.8.

$$S_a^2 = S_{Y,x}^2 \left[\frac{1}{N} + \frac{\bar{X}^2}{\Sigma (X - \bar{X})^2} \right] \quad \text{(Eq. 3.8)}$$

$$= 0.533\ (0.2 + 0.9)$$

$$= 0.586$$

Finally, test of intercept is done by Eq. 3.10.

$$t_{df} = \frac{|a - \alpha|}{\sqrt{S_a^2}} \quad \text{(Eq. 3.10)}$$

Since the $N - 2 = 3$, t_{df} calculated is t_3

$$= (2.6 - 0)/0.7659 = 3.39$$

This value (3.39) is greater than the specified t value in Appendix 2 for a degree of freedom 3. So the intercept is true and not resulted due to experimental error.

Similarly, the test for slope is to be carried out.

The variance of slope is calculated from Eq. 3.9.

$$S_b^2 = \frac{S_{Y,x}^2}{\Sigma (X - \bar{X})^2}$$

$$= (0.533)/10$$

$$= 0.0533$$

Substituting the value of S_b^2 in Eq. 3.11 we get,

$$t_3 = (2.6 - 1)/0.230 = 6.93,$$

which indicates that the slope is also real.

Stability using Linear Regression Approach

A common problem in pharmacy is fixation of expiry date based on drug degradation profile. Here the relationship of potency versus time is assumed to be linear. Usually, three batches are tested and often there is a variation in stability data between batches and also in the repeated estimations of drug potency performed at each time points. If N batches are tested for stability, while calculating intercept (initial potency) and slope of drug degradation, each time value (X) is counted N times.

Example 3: Table 3.3 given the experimental data obtained from the stability study of a formulation. If on expiry date the formulation should have 90% potency, calculate the expiry date.

Table 3.3: Potency of tablets in a stability study

Time (X) (months)	*Assay (y) (mg)*
0	26, 26, 25
3	24, 23, 25
6	22, 21, 23
9	19, 19, 20
12	17, 17, 19
18	14, 13, 15

Time (X) (months)	*Potency*			
	Batch-1 (Y_1)	*Batch-2 (Y_2)*	*Batch-3 (Y_3)*	*Average potency*
0	26	26	25	25.67
3	24	23	25	24.00
6	22	21	23	22.00
9	19	19	20	19.33
12	17	17	19	17.67
18	14	13	15	14.00
$\Sigma X = 48$	$\Sigma Y_1 = 122$	$\Sigma Y_2 = 119$	$\Sigma Y_3 = 127$	

Average of time $\bar{X} = (48 \times 3)/18 = 8$

Average of potency (sum of all values of y divided by 18)

$$\bar{Y} = (122 + 199 + 127) \div 18 = 20.44$$

Since there are three sets of Y value (potency) the time should be counted three times to calculate the average time and $X \times Y$ values. The following table is constructed accordingly.

Time (X) (months)	*Time squared (X^2)*	XY_1	XY_2	XY_3	Y_1^2	Y_2^2	Y_3^2
0	0	0	0	0	676	676	625
3	9	72	69	75	576	529	625
6	36	132	126	138	484	441	529
9	81	171	171	180	361	361	400
12	144	204	204	228	289	289	361
18	324	252	234	270	196	169	225
Summation of all the columns							
48	594	831	804	891	2582	2465	2765

Sum of time squared $\Sigma X^2 = 594 \times 3 = 1782$.

Time square has been taken 3 times because there are three sets of data.

Sum of potency squared = 2582 + 2465 + 2765 = 7812.

Sum of $\Sigma X = 48 \times 3 = 144$.

Sum of all observed values of potency $\Sigma Y = 122 + 119 + 127 = 368$.

Sum of all XY values $\Sigma XY = 831 + 804 + 891 = 2526$.

Number of X, Y pairs = 18.

It is clear from the data that concentration decreases with time and a zero order relationship $C = C_0 - Kt$ is assumed.

A and *b* can be derived from the equations and a best-fit line can be obtained as per Eq. 3.4.

$$b = \frac{N\Sigma Xy - (\Sigma X)(\Sigma y)}{N\Sigma X^2 - (\Sigma X)^2}$$

Substituting the values of

$$b = \frac{(18 \times 2526) - 144 \times 368}{18 \times 1782 - (144)^2}$$

$$b = -0.66349 \text{ mg/month}$$

$$a = \overline{Y} - b\overline{X}$$

$$= 20.44 - [(-0.66349) \times 8] = 25.75238.$$

Here, *b* represents the rate of drug degradation and is found to be –0.66349 mg/month and intercept *a*, i.e. initial potency is 25.75238 mg.

$$Y = a + bX$$

$$Y = 25.75238 - 0.66349X$$

If the tablet is usable up to 90% of the labeled potency, the value of the cutoff concentration should be 25 × 0.9 = 22.5. Substituting this value for target potency in the equation, possible expiry date of the formulation can be determined.

$$Y = 25.75238 - 0.66349X$$

$$22.5 = 25.75238 - 0.66349X$$

$$X = (22.5 - 25.75238)/-0.66349$$

$$X = 4.90 \text{ months}$$

$$\Sigma (X - \overline{X})^2 = 630.$$

$$\Sigma (y - \overline{y})^2 = 288.444$$

$$\text{Variance of } Y \text{ or } S^2_{Y,x} = \frac{\Sigma (y - \overline{y})^2 - b^2 \left[\Sigma (X - \overline{X})^2\right]}{N - 2} \quad \text{(Eq. 3.7)}$$

Using this for formula $S^2_{Y,x}$ is found to be 0.694155.

So, standard deviation of $S_{Y,x}$ = 0.83316.

Though the equation shows a clear-cut value it does not mean the true expiry date is 4.9 months. At best it is a probability that the formulation reaches 90% potency at this period. The true value of *Y* at the end of 4.9 months may be slightly greater or lesser than 90% of potency.

The range of potency at 4.9 months is given by

$$Y \pm t\left(S_{Y,x}\right)\sqrt{\frac{1}{N} + \frac{(X - \overline{X})^2}{\Sigma (X - \overline{X})^2}} \quad \text{(Eq. 3.12)}$$

Here all the values are known except t. The value of t should be obtained from the t table for the appropriate confidence coefficient. Since the value can be greater or lesser (both the sides) t value chosen should be for two-sided test. For 95% confidence, t values should be obtained from the column-head of $p = 0.975$ with degrees of freedom of $N - 2$, i.e $18 - 2 = 16$.

Hence the range of potency will be,

$$22.5 \pm 2.12 \times 0.833 \sqrt{\frac{1}{18} + \frac{(4.9 - 8)^2}{630}}$$

$$= 22.5 \pm 0.4699 \text{ mg}$$

Figure 3.1 shows that there are bands both below and above best-fit line. The band below the best-fit line reaches the target value of 90% potency in 3.5 months and the band above reaches the value much later, i.e. in 6 months. The best-fit line has the intermediate stability of 4.9 months.

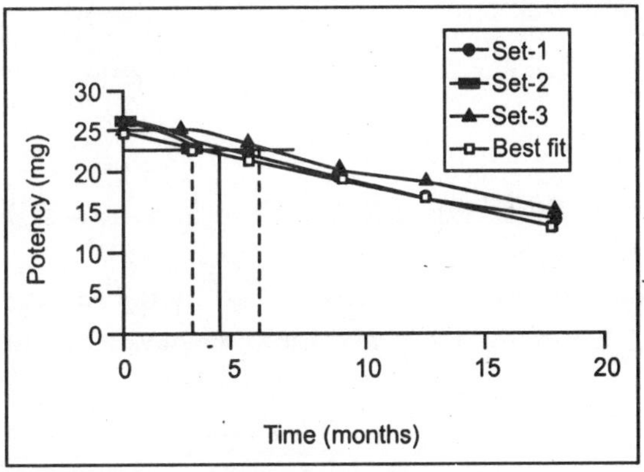

Fig. 3.1: Regression line obtained from stability data

CORRELATION

Correlation analysis investigates whether two factors (two independent variables) are related or not? For example, occurrence of cancer in an area and fruit intake of that area is two independent parameters. It is not that food intake of people is decided by their disease pattern. The occurrences of the two events, i.e. fruit consumption of an individual and his diseased state, are totally independent parameters. In correlation study, we try to investigate whether such variables are related or not. If it is found that the occurrence of cancer is less in people who take fruits regularly, we say that a negative correlation exist between fruit consumption and cancer. Here the correlation coefficient will be an indicator of reliability of that statement. The basic difference between regression and correlation is that linear regression assesses the quantitative aspect of a relationship whereas correlation investigates whether the variables are related or not? Correlation method is used to determine association of two or more variables. If the value of one variable can be predicted from knowledge of the other variable, we say the variables are correlated. The stronger the correlation, better is the prediction. If we could predict the dissolution time of the tablet from the thickness of its coating, we say the two variables (coating thickness and dissolution time) are correlated.

Correlation analysis assumes linear relationship between two variables. Correlation is usually depicted as scatter plots. In this, data are represented as pairs (X, Y) with the objective of demonstrating a trend or relationship between the X, Y variables.

A positive slope indicates positive correlation and negative slope, a negative relationship.

Sometimes, relationship between two variables is not obvious. It may be camouflaged because of variability. Correlation analysis may reveal the relation between factors. However, a strong correlation between two variables does not indicate cause and effect relationship.

Correlation Coefficient

Correlation coefficient is a measure or indicator of the degree of correlation but it is not a measure of linearity. A strong correlation does not mean that the relationship between *X* and *Y* is straight line. Correlation coefficient is indicated by symbol *r*.

$$r = \frac{\Sigma(X-\bar{X})(y-\bar{y})}{\sqrt{\Sigma(X-\bar{X})^2 - \Sigma(y-\bar{y})^2}} \quad \text{(Eq. 3.13)}$$

r^2 represents the relative reduction in the sum of square of the variable *y*, resulting from the fitting of *X* and *y* line. Sometimes, the symbol R^2 is also used in the statistical packages.

The concept can be clarified by taking an example.

Suppose, *X* and *y* values collected from a population are as follows (Table 3.4):

Table 3.4: Study of correlation between *X* and *Y*

X	y	Xy
0	0	0
2	2	4
4	10	40

First the slope is determined.

$\Sigma X = 0 + 2 + 4 = 6$

$\Sigma Y = 0 + 2 + 10 = 12$

$\Sigma X^2 = 2^2 + 4^2 + 0 = 20$

$\Sigma XY = 0 + 4 + 40 = 44$

$\bar{X} = (0 + 2 + 4)/3 = 2$

$\bar{Y} = (0 + 2 + 10)/3 = 4$

N = Number of *X*, *y* pair is 3.

As per Eq. 3.4

$$b = \frac{N\Sigma Xy - (\Sigma X)(\Sigma y)}{N\Sigma X^2 - (\Sigma X)^2} \quad \text{(Eq. 3.4)}$$

$$b = \frac{3 \times 44 - 6 \times 12}{3 \times 20 - 6^2} = 2.5$$

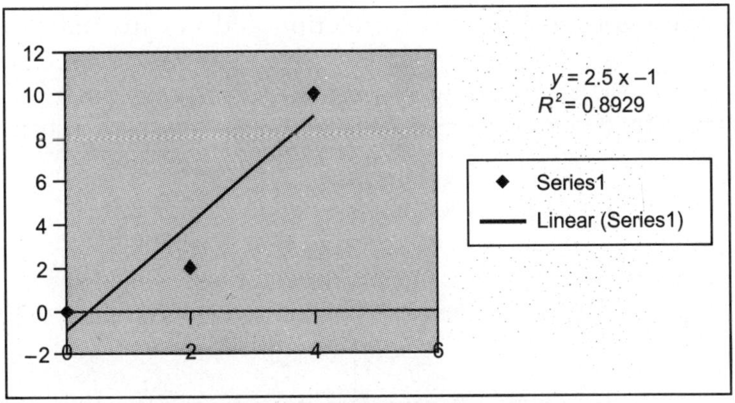

Fig. 3.2: Best-fit line from data in Table 3.3

Now to determine the extent of association or correlation coefficient, we have to determine the correlation coefficient r.

Correlation coefficient 'r' is the square root of relative reduction of the sum of the squares of Y.

The sum of squares due to deviation of the y values is $\Sigma (y - \bar{y})^2$.

Due to fitting $\Sigma (y - \bar{y})^2$, i.e. sum of squares was reduced by $b^2 [\Sigma (X - \bar{X})^2]$, the difference is $\Sigma (y - \bar{y})^2 - [\Sigma (X - \bar{X})^2]$.

In the given problem

$$\Sigma (X - \bar{X})^2 = 2^2 + 0 + 2^2 = 8$$

$$\Sigma (y - \bar{y})^2 = 4^2 + 2^2 + 6^2 = 56$$

$$b = 2.5$$

The reduction in the sum of squares is $56 - (2.5)^2 \times 8 = 6$.

The original sum of square of y was 56, which was reduced to 6 because of fitting. The overall reduction is $56 - 6 = 50$. r^2 is the relative reduction of the sum of the squares. Relative reduction $r^2 = 50/56 = 0.893$ or $r = 0.945$.

Accordingly, r can be interpreted as the relative degree of scatter about the regression line. If X, Y values lie exactly on a straight line, i.e. variance of Y is zero, and r equal to ± 1. Perfect positive relationship is indicated when value of r is 1 whereas -1 indicates perfect negative relationship. If the value of correlation coefficient is found to be '0' it confirms that there is no relationship between X and Y.

Correlation Vs Regression

In correlation study, X and Y both are independent variables. In contrast, in linear regression, X represents an independent variable while Y is a function of X.

In regression analysis the basic assumption is that, X and Y are linearly correlated.

On the other hand, statistical test of correlation is a test for correlation or independence. The correlation coefficient actually estimates the degree of closeness of a linear relation between two variables Y and X.

Test of Zero Correlation

The correlation coefficients are determined from sample data (X, Y pair). So there is a question whether an observed correlation coefficient is real or due to chance.

When we analyze the data from totally unrelated sources, random variation can result in a finite value of correlation coefficient rather than zero. For this, observed correlation coefficient r is tested against a hypothetical value of H_0. This test is a t test with ($N - 2$) degree of freedom. Y is assumed to be a normal variable.

The null hypothesis assumes there is no correlation and is written as H_0: $\rho = 0$, here ρ denotes the true correlation coefficient. The alternative hypothesis is H_a: $\rho \neq 0$.

$$t_{N-2} = \frac{\left| r\sqrt{N-2} \right|}{\sqrt{1-r^2}} \qquad \text{(Eq. 3.14)}$$

The calculated value of t_{N-2} obtained is referred to as t distribution with ($N - 2$) degrees of freedom, where N is the sample size. If the calculated value of t is greater than referred value of t, the null hypothesis is rejected and correlation between X and Y is established. This test is analogous to the test of significance for slope in regression analysis.

MULTIPLE LINEAR REGRESSION ANALYSIS

Multiple regression analysis is an extension of linear regression in which a response is related to more than one independent variable. Linear regression has the general formula: $Y = A + BX$.

In multiple regression, the number of variables is more, so the expression is:

$$Y = B_0 + B_iX_i + \ldots\ldots B_nX_n \qquad \text{(Eq. 3.15)}$$

Where,

Y is the dependent variable.

X_i is the ith independent variable.

B_i is the regression coefficient for the ith variable.

Multiple regression analysis is carried out to quantify the relationship between a response (dependent variable) and a number of independent variables by means of an equation. For example, tablet disintegration may be a function of many variables such as level of disintegrant, binder and lubricants. So, to predict the disintegration time, a multiple regression equation can be used. The generalized expression is:

$$Y = B_0 + B_1X_1 + B_2X_2 + B_3X_3 \ldots\ldots$$

The coefficients B_1, B_2 and B_3 correspond to the slope (B) in linear regression. B_0 is the intercept. Unlike linear regression, this equation cannot be depicted on two-dimensional plane. When the number of independent variables is two (X_1 and X_2), the response can be depicted as a surface in three-dimensional diagram (Fig. 3.3). But when the number of variables is more than two, it is not possible to graph the response in two dimensions.

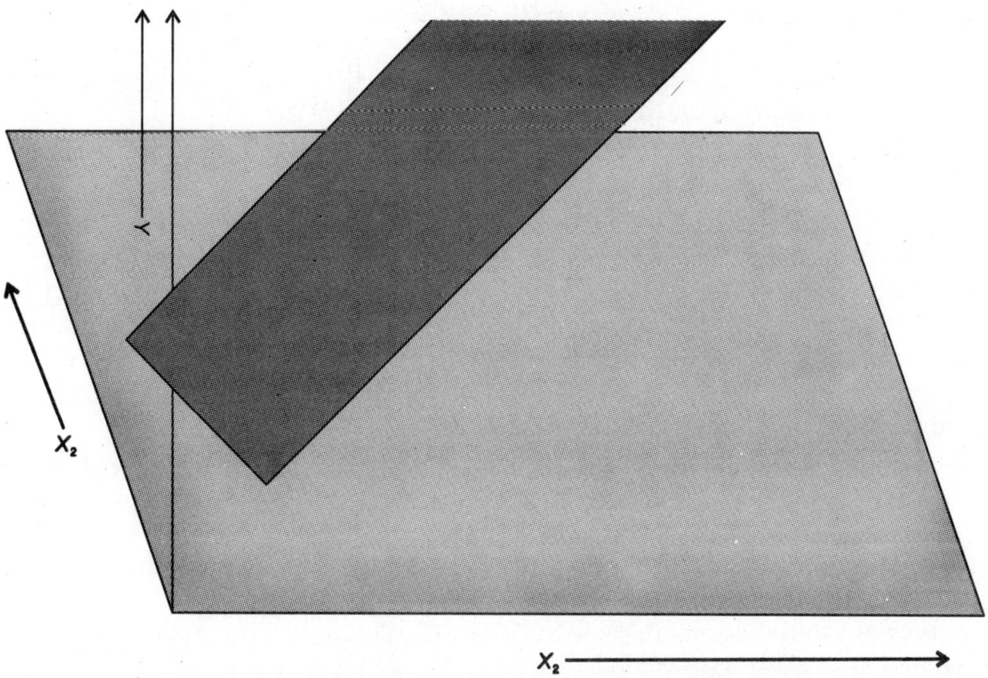

Fig. 3.3: A three-dimensional representation of multiple regression equation response

Data obtained from factorial experiments are often used to construct multiple regression equation. In 2^3 factorials, there are three factors, but interaction of factors may also affect the response.

In multiple regression equations, interactions are represented by cross-product terms such as $X_1 X_2$ or $X_1 X_2 X_3$. Only the terms, which have meaningful effect, are included into the equation. Multiple regression analysis is lengthy and time-consuming. With the increased availability of computer and specialist softwares, hand analysis is done only as a learning tool to gain insight into the process.

Utility of Multiple Regression Analysis in Pharmacy

In linear regression we have seen that, if we have only two data pairs of *X*, *Y*, both the parameters (slope and intercept) will be fixed because only one specific line can be drawn through them. But if more than two points are there, the best-fit line is drawn on the basis of statistical analysis. The best-fit line so obtained accommodates all the *X*, *Y* pairs observed in a study. Similarly, when a response is a function of a number of factors it is difficult to ascertain the contribution of an individual factor to the overall response. A detailed statistical analysis is required to find out the contribution of each factor to the overall response.

For example, the activity of a drug molecule may be doubled by the presence of OH groups and reduced by NH_2 group and disappear totally if a certain group is not there. Multiple regression analysis is performed to find out the individual contribution of these factors with respect to the overall effect. In real life pharmaceutical problems, actual number of unknown variables is countless. Data for multiple regressions may come from factorial designs. Data from undesigned experiments may also be analyzed by multiple regression analysis.

The Basic Principle of Multiple Correlations

It is known that if we have two equations containing the same unknown variables X and Y, the value of the individual factors can be derived by the process of gradual elimination. To construct a linear model relating a response Y, with one or more independent variables (X_i), the number of observations should be equal to or greater than the number of parameters to be estimated, i.e. number of coefficients to be determined.

Concept of Developing Predictive Equation

To have some idea of this concept, let us try to develop a predictive model of activity with 4 variables; where overall effect of a drug is affected by NH_2, COOH, OH and an aromatic ring. We will use the symbol X_1, X_2, X_3, X_4 for NH_2, COOH, OH and the aromatic ring respectively. The intensity of the therapeutic response is denoted by numerical value (0, indicating no activity and 100, the strongest activity). For simplification, let us assume that we have 4 molecules and all the molecules have all the groups in varying proportion.

The generalized activity equation is

$$Y = B_1X_1 + B_2X_2 + B_3X_3 + B_4X_4 \qquad \text{(Eq. 3.16)}$$

Where B_1, B_2, B_3 and B_4 are the coefficients (in this case, the power or contribution to therapeutic effect is by a single unit of a group of X_1, X_2, X_3, X_4).

So if a molecule contains one unit of each moiety, i.e. X_1, X_2, X_3, X_4, its overall therapeutic activity will be obtained by substituting 1 in the generalized equation.

$$Y = B_1(1) + B_2(1) + B_3(1) + B_4(1)$$

$$Y = B_1 + B_2 + B_3 + B_4$$

Where, Y represents the overall activity and B_1, B_2, B_3 and B_4 are the coefficients of the groups.

If a set of such molecules are generated with known number of therapeutically active groups and experimentally derived activity, the power of each group can be obtained by generating a set of equations and gradually eliminating factors. Finally, a predictive polynomial equation can be generated using power of factors as coefficients.

Let us assume that four such molecules and their experimentally derived activity are represented by:

$$B_1 + B_2 + B_3 + B_4 = 24 \qquad (i)$$

$$B_1 + 2B_2 + 2B_3 + 2B_4 = 28 \qquad (ii)$$

$$B_1 + B_2 + B_3 + 3B_4 = 34 \qquad (iii)$$

$$2B_1 + B_2 + 3B_3 + B_4 = 40 \qquad (iv)$$

To determine the coefficients, we have to consider all the equations and eliminate the variables sequentially.

First to eliminate B_1,

The coefficients of B_1 in all the equations are brought to the same value. The coefficients of B_1 are 1, 1, 1, 2 and the LCM is 2.

By multiplying equations (*i*), (*ii*), (*iii*) with this LCM, i.e. 2, we get,

$$2B_1 + 2B_2 + 2B_3 + 2B_4 = 48 \quad (v)$$
$$2B_1 + 4B_2 + 4B_3 + 4B_4 = 56 \quad (vi)$$
$$2B_1 + 2B_2 + 2B_3 + 6B_4 = 68 \quad (vii)$$

By subtracting Eq. (*v*) from Eq. (*vi*) we get,

$$2B_2 + 2B_3 + 2B_4 = 8$$

Or, $$B_2 + B_3 + B_4 = 4 \quad (viii)$$

Similarly, by subtracting Eq. (*vi*) from Eq. (*vii*), we get

$$-2B_2 - 2B_3 + 2B_4 = 12$$
$$-B_2 - B_3 + B_4 = 6 \quad (ix)$$

By adding Eqs (*viii*) and (*ix*) we get,

$$2B_4 = 10$$

Or, $$B_4 = 5 \quad (x)$$

Similarly, by subtracting Eq. (*iv*) from Eq. (*vii*) we get,

$$B_2 - B_3 + 5B_4 = 28 \quad (xi)$$

Adding Eqs (*viii*) and (*xi*) we get,

$$2B_2 + 6B_4 = 32$$

Or, $$B_2 + 3B_4 = 16 \quad (xii)$$

Substituting $B_4 = 5$, the value of B_2 is found to be 1

$$B_2 = 1 \quad (xiii)$$

Once the values of both B_2 and B_4 are substituted in Eq. (*xi*) the value of B_3 can be found.

$$B_2 - B_3 + 5B_4 = 28$$
$$1 - B_3 + 5 \times 5 = 28$$
$$B_3 = -2$$

Similarly, the value of B_1 can be obtained from any of the equations:

$$B_1 + B_2 + B_3 + B_4 = 24 \quad (i)$$
$$B_1 + 1 - 2 + 5 = 24$$
$$B_1 = 20$$

So ultimately the generalized expression becomes

$$Y = 20X_1 + X_2 - 2X_3 + 5X_4$$

If there are M parameters (coefficients) in the regression model, M observations will result in an exact fit. In our example, there were 4 coefficients and only 4 observations were made.

However, if we had more than four observations, i.e. greater than the number of parameters (M), coefficients would be calculated in such a way as to minimize the squared deviations of the observations from the least squares regression fit. The relationship of the independent variables and the dependent variables must be linear in order to obtain a regression equation.

The X_i can be a non-linear function, (e.g. $Y = X^2$, or log X) but coefficients cannot be non-linear function. The basic problem in multiple regression analysis lies in the estimation of errors and coefficients of the regression model. When many independent variables are entered into a regression equation only significant or meaningful terms are retained.

In designed experiments, significance of each term is determined by ANOVA. In undesigned experiments, independent variables are often related. For example, two groups or substituents may occur always together.

If two variables are highly correlated, the inclusion of them into the regression equation is unnecessary. However, there is no hard and fast rule whether these variables should be included or not.

Usually, there are a number of methods to address this problem. One method involves regression fits with all possible constructions. If two variables are there, 2^2 number of effects are possible. They are:

1. $Y = B_0$ (here X_1 and X_2 both have no effect).
2. $Y = B_0 + B_1X_1$ (only X_1 has effect).
3. $Y = B_0 + B_2X_2$ (only X_2 has effect).
4. $Y = B_0 + B_1X_1 + B_2X_2$ (both X_1 and X_2 influence the outcome).

The best equation may be selected based on the fit (activity predicted by the coefficients is compared with actual response and evaluated for closeness of the response).

The multiple correlation coefficient r^2 is a measure of the fit. It is the sum of the squares due to regression divided by sum of the squares without regression. If with 3 variables we get a regression of 0.9 and with 4 variables we get a regression of 0.91, then it is better to omit the fourth variable because inclusion increases the accuracy of prediction marginally but equation becomes comparatively bulky.

The second method is the popular stepwise procedure. In this, independent variables are entered into the equation one at a time starting with the variable, which has the highest correlation with the dependent variable.

Multiple regression equations are models of real systems, which can at best be an approximation of reality. Coefficients can give insights into the mechanism of a process. However, error, i.e. variability in the estimation of the coefficients, extrapolating to areas outside the level of variables in the experiment, can affect the reliability of the predicted value.

BIBLIOGRAPHY

1. De Muth James E, *Basic Statistics and Pharmaceutical Statistical Applications*, Marcel Dekker, Inc, 1999.
2. Draper NR and Smith H., *Applied Regression Analysis*, Second edition, Wiley and Sons, 1981.
3. Sanford Bolton, *Practical and Clinical Applications*, Third edition, Marcel Dekker, Inc, 1997.
4. Snedector GW and Cochran WG., *Statistical Methods*, Eighth edition, Iowa State University Press, 1989.

4 Factorial Design

INTRODUCTION

Factorial designs are used in experiments where effects of different factors on experimental results are to be elucidated. When several factors are present in one product, they may affect the response individually and also in combination. In pharmaceutical dosage forms, many ingredients exist together. Even if a formulation designer takes precaution to ensure that the excipients do not affect the clinical responses of drugs, the physical parameters of dosage forms, e.g. dissolution time, hardness, etc. are often affected. So, now-a-days, instead of the traditional trial and error methods, formulation development is done according to some set guidelines. This chapter introduces factorial design which is currently the design of choice for product development in pharmaceutical industries.

What is Factorial Design?

While designing a drug product, little flexibility exists in the choice of quantity and quality of the active ingredients, but the level of excipients can be altered to generate desirable pharmaceutical parameters. Pharmacopoeias prescribe standards for specific dosage forms, which must be met for gaining official approval. So there is compelling official and commercial need to select and use the ingredients in optimized proportion to produce quality products within the given set of constraints. Initially industries depended only on experience but now the concepts of formulation development have changed and guidelines have evolved to come up with optimized formula through logical designing. Factorial design is one such method for designing experiments that generate enough data to develop predictive models, on the basis of which an optimized product can be developed. It can elucidate the effect of a single ingredient or its interactive effect, when simultaneously used along with a number of other components. Factorial designs are orthogonal, i.e. the response is thought to be due to the effect of experimental variables only. It is considered to be free of other factors.

If *A*, *B* and *C* are the 3 factors chosen for the experiment and each is tested at 2 levels, the experiment is called 2^3 experiment. The total number of experiments in factorial design (where all the factors are tested at the same number of levels) is given by exponential expression where the base is equivalent to the number of levels and the power represents the number of factors.

There may be factors in a product, which may influence the outcome but not relevant to the experiment. Such factors should be kept constant. Apart from the pharmaceutical/pharmacological factors, variations in response can occur from instrumental and personal errors too. The more the control of extraneous factors, the smaller will be the residual variation. The residual error is the random error remaining after ANOVA removes the variability due to factors and their interactions.

Advantages of Factorial Experiment

The results of a properly conducted factorial experiment can be used to determine many effects.

1. Factorial design can help to interpret the mechanism of an experimental system.
2. Factorial design can help us to select a particular condition or a set of conditions as the most suitable under the given constraints.
3. Factorial designs can also be used as guidelines for further experiments.

Symbols used in Factorial Experiments

The objective of a factorial experiment is to characterize the effect of change in the levels of a factor or combinations of factors on the overall response. If the aim of the experiment is to determine the effect of a diluent at 2 levels on the dissolution time of a tablet, only two experiments will be required, provided other factors are constant. Similarly, if the dose of drug and diluents are each tested at two levels, a 2-factor 2-level (2^2) experiment will be required (Table 4.1). Usually, codes are assigned to indicate the experiments when number of experiments is large. For example, if the drug is taken as a factor, placebo (dosage form with no drug) will be considered as a composition with the low level of that factor (drug). The total number of experiments in factorial design includes combination of all levels and all factors. For investigating the effect of drug concentration and disintegrant concentration on dissolution of a tablet, both the factors need to be tested at both the levels. Hence, 2^n ($n = 2$) or 4 experiments will be required.

There are some fixed norms followed for coding the experiments. Let A be the symbol assigned to drug and B to the disintegrant.

When all factors are at low levels the experiment is coded as 1.

When A is at high level but B is at low level it is coded as a.

When A is at low level but B is at high level it is coded as b.

When both are at high levels the symbol is ab.

Table 4.1: Design for a 2^2 factorial experiment

S. no.	*Formulation*	*Symbol*
1	Low drug + Low disintegrant	1
2	High drug + Low disintegrant	*a*
3	Low drug + High disintegrant	*b*
4	High drug + High disintegrant	*ab*

Coding: When the factors present in a formulation, are in low concentration, the code used is minus (–) and when factors are in high concentration, the code used is plus (+).

Some Common Terms used in Factorial Experiments

Factor: This term indicates assigned variables, e.g. type of an excipient, temperature of processing, time, etc.

Factors can be both qualitative and quantitative in nature. Examples of the quantitative factors are—Analysts employed, types of lubricants, or method selected whereas percent of additives used in a formulation is a quantitative factor. Single factor designs are comparable to one-way ANOVA designs. An experimental design to compare 3 drugs, using different patients in each group is a one-way design with the single factor (drug).

Level: Levels indicate number of values or designations assigned to a factor. Temperature is a factor whereas 30°C and 50°C are the 2 levels of this factor. Similarly, if concentration of an excipient is considered as a factor, different concentrations, (e.g. 0.1% and 0.5%) will be the levels.

Independent variable: These are the factors, which can be changed by the developer at will, e.g. mixing time. A developer can increase or decrease the time of mixing as per his will.

Dependent variable: The response of the independent variables is dependent variable.

Interaction: Lack of additivity is called interaction. Often the effect of one factor may be modified by the presence of other factors. Let us assume that in a tablet, factor *A* can cause a delay in dissolution by 5 minutes and factor *B* by 7 minutes. On being used together, if they cause a delay of 12 minutes (5 minutes due to *A* + 7 minutes due to *B*), they are said to have additive effects. Any deviation from this value is interaction. A higher effect (e.g. the dissolution time of 20 minutes) is synergistic and a lower effect (e.g. 9 minutes) is antagonistic interaction. As factorial experiments consist of all combinations of all levels of all factors, these interactions can be evaluated by analyzing the results of experiments.

Effects: Effect of a factor is defined as the change in response caused by varying the level of factors. The main effect of a factor is the effect averaged over all of the other factors. In a two-factor experiment with two levels each of drug and disintegrant, the main effect of drug would be the difference between the average response of the drug at high level (i.e. *a* and *ab*) and the average response of the drug at low level (i.e. 1 and *b*).

Therefore, main effect of drug would be $(a + ab - 1 - b)/2$.

If an experiment is carried out using three levels of an ingredient while other factors are constant and the responses obtained are plotted against the levels of that factor, the concentration-response profile may either be linear or curved (quadratic). If no interaction occurs, the main effects can be efficiently estimated by simple experimentation (using two levels only). In case of interactions, factorial designs are necessary to identify the main effects.

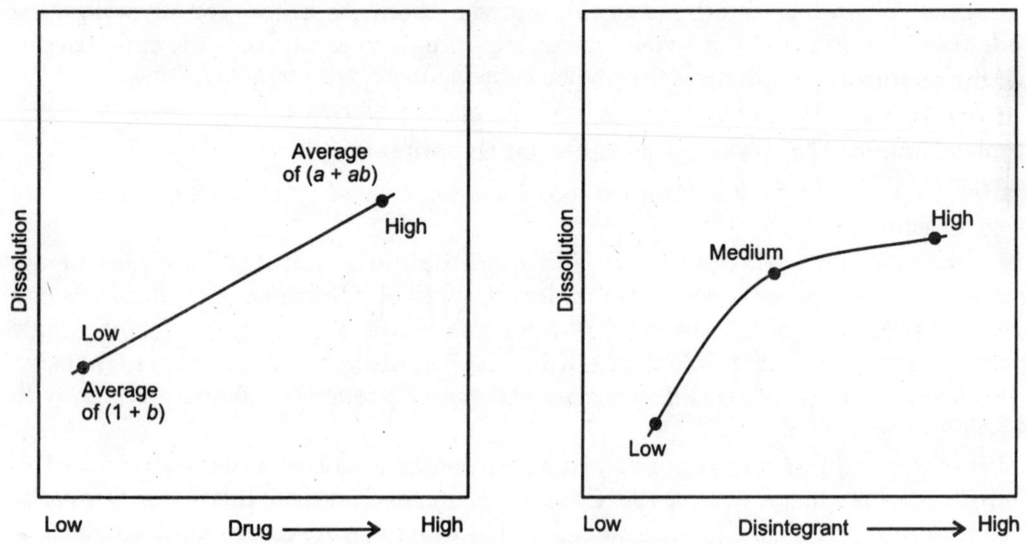

Fig. 4.1: The effect of drug and disintegrant concentration on dissolution time

Figure 4.1 depicts the effect of drug and disintegrant concentration on dissolution time of a tablet. The first one (drug) shows a linear profile as only two levels are tested. In the second one (disintegrant) three levels of disintegrant are used and a curved profile is obtained.

In the first case, the main effect can be characterized as a linear response since the effect is the difference between only two points. But practically, we need more than two points, where the response profile is non-linear. In the second graph, the levels of disintegrant are plotted against time of dissolution (response) and a curve is obtained. Hence, the main effect is less clear.

Guidelines for Designing

If factors are quantitative, two or more levels are chosen. If a response is known to be a linear function of a factor, two levels are sufficient. If the response is known to be non-linear, at least 3 levels are required to characterize the response. A rule of thumb for fixing the levels of an ingredient is usually used in two-level experiments. It divides the extreme ranges of a factor into four equal parts and take one-fourth and three-fourth values as the choice of levels.

Suppose, an excipient is allowed to be used in the range of 0 to 8% concentration.

$$\text{Range} = (8 - 0) = 8\%$$

The lower level chosen for factorial experiments would be one-fourth of the range.

$$\frac{8\% \times 1}{4} = 2\%$$

The higher level would be three-fourths of the range, i.e.

$$\frac{8\% \times 3}{4} = 6\%$$

If the factors are qualitative, the choice is predefined (type of analysts).

If one factor were to be tested at 3 levels and other two at two levels, the total number of experiments would be $2 \times 2 \times 3 = 12$. The trials of factorial design should be done in random order to avoid bias.

A Worked Example of 2^3 Factorial Experiment

To clarify the concept, let us think of an experiment where the effect of three factors drug, disintegrant and lubricant on the dissolution time of tablets, is to be evaluated. We name these factors as *A*, *B* and *C*. Since, 3 factors are simultaneously evaluated, total number of experiments needed is 2^3 where 2 represents the level and 3 the number of factors.

The levels chosen for drug are –0 (placebo) and 50, for disintegrant 0 and 20 and for lubricant 0 and 1 mg respectively. By convention in two-level experiments, the low levels are coded as minus (–) and high levels as plus (+). The response variable is the dissolution time. The combination of factors and the experimental results can be tabulated as in Table 4.2.

Table 4.2: Dissolution time obtained at various combinations of factors

Combination	*Drug (A)*	*Disintegrant (B)*	*Lubricant (C)*	*Dissolution time (Y)*
1	–	–	–	20
a	+	–	–	24
b	–	+	–	18
ab	+	+	–	21
c	–	–	+	40
ac	+	–	+	43
bc	–	+	+	37
abc	+	+	+	39

When three factors are involved, response may be affected by all the three factors individually as well as by their interactions.

So the interactions possible are of four types; namely *ab* (*A* interacting with *B*), *ac* (*A* interacting with *C*), *bc* (*B* interacting with *C*) and *abc*, where *A*, *B* and *C* all interact and affect the response due to the formation of a complex interaction factor. The interaction factors may contribute either positively or negatively to a particular response. The response is the sum of seven types of responses if all types of interactions take place. The first formulation (formulation code 1) has all three factors in the negative level; hence response of this formulation is assumed to be the effect of ingredients other than factors tested. The computation of the main effects is done from the results by performing ANOVA or using simple calculators.

In the manual calculation, the first step is arranging the information in tabular form that would accommodate all types of effects. A table is constructed by placing the sign (+/–) in each column (*A*, *B*, *C* and their every possible interaction, i.e. *AB*, *AC*, *BC*, *ABC*). Interaction factors are assigned sign by multiplying the signs of individual factors. In formulation 1, all 3 factors have negative sign. So *AB*, the product of 2 negative signs, is positive. Similarly, result of multiplication of 3 negative signs, *ABC*, has a negative sign in the first row. Table 4.3 shows an example of factor combinations and experimental results using such coded signs.

Table 4.3: Signs of the various interaction factors

Combination	*(A)*	*(B)*	*(C)*	*AB*	*AC*	*BC*	*ABC*	*Y (minutes)*
1	–	–	–	+	+	+	–	20
a	+	–	–	–	–	+	+	24
b	–	+	–	–	+	–	+	18
ab	+	+	–	+	–	–	–	21
c	–	–	+	+	–	–	+	40
ac	+	–	+	–	+	–	–	43
bc	–	+	+	–	–	+	–	37
abc	+	+	+	+	+	+	+	39

Calculation of the Effects

In each column, there are 8 entries out of which 4 have +ve sign and the remaining 4 have –ve sign. To calculate the average effects of each of the seven factors (3 main effects *A*, *B*, *C* and 4 interaction effects) the responses should be multiplied by the signs of the respective columns and added. Finally, the result should be divided by 2^{n-1}. So in this case, the total is divided by 2^{3-1} or 4.

Calculation of the Effect of A

First, the values in response column are multiplied with the signs under the column-head *A*.

Next, the values are added.

Finally, the total is divide by 4.

$$(-20 + 24 - 18 + 21 - 40 + 43 - 37 + 39) = 12.$$

The main effect of *A* is 12/4 = 3.

The value is 3 and sign of this value is positive. This indicates the effect of increasing the drug concentration from low to high level is prolongation of the dissolution time by 3 minutes.

Similarly, for *B* the total is,

$$(-20 - 24 + 18 + 21 - 40 - 43 + 37 + 39) = -12$$

Divided by 4, the value is –3, which is the net effect of increasing the disintegrant concentration. The dissolution time is reduced by 3 minutes due to increase in disintegrant concentration.

For C the total is,

$$(-20 - 24 - 18 - 21 + 40 + 43 + 37 + 39) = 76.$$

Divided by 4 the value comes out as 19, which indicates the main effect of C or effect of increasing the lubricant concentration. Here, the dissolution time is extended by 19 minutes.

Similarly, the interaction factors can be calculated from this data.

The total for the column AB is (20 – 24 – 18 + 21 + 40 – 43 – 37 + 39) = –2. Hence, –2/4 or –0.5 is negative contribution of AB to total dissolution time. This indicates interaction between drug and disintegrant takes place but the effect is very small. It minimally reduces the dissolution time (0.5 minutes).

Analysis of the Results

As told before, like every experiment, there are chances of mistakes in the factorial experiments too. ANOVA is used to ascertain the reliability of the result. Factorial designs are elaborate and computers are used for data analysis. However, for simple experiments, the method devised by Yates et al. can be used if the levels of the factors are limited to 2.

In Yates method, the data is arranged in standard order followed by addition and subtraction in pairs. If the number of factors is N, the process of summation and subtraction is done repeatedly to create N columns. In the given example, there are 3 factors, so 3 columns are created. The 4th column is obtained by dividing the 3rd column with 2^{n-1}, i.e. 4. The value in this column (4th) shows the mean effects. Finally, the 5th column is created by squaring the values of 3rd column and dividing it by 2^n, i.e. 8, the values in this column represent the mean square variance of a factor interaction.

Table 4.4: Yates analysis of the factorial experiment for analysis of variance

Formulation	*Response*	*Column (1)*	*Column (2)*	*Column (3)*	*Effect (3)/4*	*MSV* (3)²/8*
1	20	44	83	242	60.5	–
a	24	39	159	12	3	18
b	18	83	7	–12	–3	18
ab	21	76	5	–2	–0.5	0.5
c	40	4	–5	76	19	722
ac	43	3	–7	–2	–0.5	0.5
bc	37	3	–1	–2	–0.5	0.5
abc	39	2	–1	0	0.0	0.0

*MSV = mean square variance is obtained by squaring the values of nth column (3rd column) and dividing it by 2^n, i.e. 8.

In Table 4.4, a specific order is followed in the addition and subtraction. Note that, while adding values are taken from top to bottom (1 + a), (b + ab), (c + ac), (bc + abc). While subtracting it is always bottom minus top, i.e. (a – 1), (ab – b), (ac – c), etc.

Interpretation of Results

The results of experiments are typically presented in ANOVA table (Table 4.5). In 2^n factorial, each effect and interaction has 1 degree of freedom. To get the F value, we need to divide the mean square variance by the error mean square. To minimize error, replicate experiments are needed but replication increases the total number of experiments. So it can be taken from previous experiences. However, in large experiments, the error can be estimated by pooling the mean squares from higher order interactions. In the present tableting experiment, errors can be taken from the mean square corresponding to the two-way interactions *AB*, *AC*, *BC* and *ABC* (a three-way interaction). The values of these interactions are taken to be 0 from prior experiences. In other words, based on the knowledge of separate experiments, we know that these factors do not interact with each other and hence should have an effect of 0. However, Table 4.4 indicates there is some minimal effect for these interactions too. So these variance values obtained can be taken to be errors. The total error here when no interaction is present, is given by sum of the values obtained for *AB*, *AC*, *BC*, *ABC*. The variance of *ABC* is 0, so, the mean estimate of error is (0.5 + 0.5 + 0.5)/3 = 0.5.

F value for *A* is 18/0.5 = 36.

For *B* too, this value is 36.

Table 4.5: ANOVA table for various factors

Source	*Degree of freedom*	*Mean square variance*	$F^{1/3}$
A	1	18	36
B	1	18	36
C	1	722	1444
Residual	3	0.5	

For C the value is 722/0.5 = 1444.

In the *F* table for 95% confidence level (Appendix 3), we can see the *F* value for d.f. 1/3, i.e. the value under the column-head 1 in the row number 3. Since this value for *F* is 10.1, all *A*, *B* and *C* are considered to have significant effects on tablet dissolution time. Influence of C is the highest and beyond doubt it prolongs the process to the greatest degree.

BIBLIOGRAPHY

1. Davies OL, The design and analysis of industrial experiments, Hafner New York, 1963.
2. De, Muth James E, Basic statistics and pharmaceutical statistical applications, Marcel Dekker, Inc, 1999.
3. Sanford Bolton, *Practical and Clinical Applications*, Third edition, Marcel Dekker, Inc, 1997.

5 Optimization Techniques

INTRODUCTION

Development of a pharmaceutical formulation is a lengthy process. It involves enormous cost in terms of man, material and time. Making the right choice of ingredients and subjecting them to the right processes to come up with products that are best and reproducible within the given set of conditions or constraints is a formidable task.

Before introducing the drug products into market for public consumption, pharmaceutical industries need to follow certain norms. They should produce concrete proof that the product is safe and beneficial for the patients. Process and product reproducibility is a basic need to assure the drug approval. For a new drug or formulation to be approved by the authorities, the manufacturer must submit development reports. Initially, industries relied on experience. Till the recent era, formulation design was considered as 'Art' rather than a 'Science'. Formulation design in a planned and systematic manner was considered to be a job, reserved for the experts only. Recently, there has been a change in this attitude and statistics have found use in the designing of pharmaceutical products. Optimization, a new approach that uses the concept of statistics to optimize the formulation and process parameters, is being increasingly used in formulation designing. This chapter introduces some basic concepts of optimization.

The new approach has several advantages over the traditional trial-error method. It follows certain well-established guidelines and even an inexperienced worker can develop a formulation based on these guidelines. A clear-cut goal is set and experimental formulations are compared against these set objectives. By proper planning and logical reasoning number of experiments can be reduced, which reduces the cost.

The optimization operation involves series of logical steps. In general, the optimization problems can be classified into two categories.

1. Constrained
2. Unconstrained.

In pharmacy, we usually have constrained problems. Optimized formulations must comply with some preselected results. For example, a tablet must dissolve within a certain time and release the active ingredients. The ideal time within which it should dissolve is a preselected parameter. Similarly, the ideal hardness, which makes the tablet withstand the rigors of handling and transportation, is another prefixed parameter. Optimization process is undertaken to produce formulations that satisfy these given set of conditions to a maximum degree within the given constraints.

Development of a dosage form is a multi-step process. In a formulation, the quality and quantity of certain ingredients are unchangeable and hence considered as fixed parameter. In a formulation, often the quantity of drug is fixed. Official books like pharmacopoeias decide its standard of purity. But a wide choice is available to the method developer in terms of excipients. The first step of method development is choice of excipient, where a few ideal excipients out of many available have to be chosen. Preformulation studies are carried out to find the possible incompatibilities and excipients, which are compatible with the drug.

The second part is design or making of a formula to decide the percentage of each excipient to come up with the desired drug product. Official restraints like percent of preservatives or antioxidants allowed and cost considerations are the usual constraints of this step. In most of the cases, series of experimental formulations are made and analyzing these experimental formulations, the final formula is developed.

The third step is processing. Processing is also done in steps:

(*a*) Selection of process

(*b*) Setting the timings and intensity parameters, etc. of a process.

Statistical optimization is a broad guideline used in the formulation design to obtain a targeted product (or a product closest to the target) within the given set of constraints. In short, it refers to the quantitative techniques of this formulation design and processing. Several designs have been proposed for this but the basic principle is changing of a single factor while keeping all others constant. It helps to find the effect of that factor on the overall response, which is a composite parameter.

SOME IMPORTANT DEFINITIONS

Factors: Factors are independent variables, which can be directly controlled by the formulator, e.g. quantity of diluent, mixing time, etc.

Response: Response is a dependent variable. The value of response changes with the changes in the levels of factors, which are independent variables. If there is only one variable, the relationship between cause (independent variable) and effect (dependent variable) can be displayed on a plain two-dimensional graph. But if the response is the outcome of two variables, a three-dimensional graph is required which comes in the form of response surface.

Contour plots: A hill range is the best approximation of contour plot in real life. Ordinary plots are two-dimensional. Here, we can see the changes in *Y*-axis against the different values of *X*-axis. But when more than two parameters are involved, a planar plot cannot represent the response profile. For example, we may have practical data that an emulsion prepared at 1000 rpm for the duration of 5 and 10 minutes results in 30 minutes and 1-hour cracking time but if time of rotation is 1 minute it cracks within 5 minutes. So we can only show it if cracking time (response due to composite parameter of rpm and rotation time) is shown as elevations over a surface. Suppose, the cracking time of 5 minutes is represented by an elevation of 1 mm. A slanting graph starting at Y-axis value of 1000 rpm elevated 1 mm at 1 minute point and elevated 6 and 12 mm at 5 and 10 minute points would give a three-dimensional graph which would look like a series of hilltops. If all these hilltops are joined, it looks like a slanted surface. This surface can be analyzed to find the optimum values for the optimum rpm and rotation time for a stable formulation.

Statistical methods used in optimization are usually of two types:

1. ***Evolutionary operations:*** In this, experiment continues as optimization proceeds.
2. ***Search methods:*** Here, responses of the different compositions are ascertained first and analyzed for effect of individual factors. Analysis is done after experiment is complete. The cause-effect relationship is determined by the statistical analysis of experimental data.

Classical optimization uses calculus, where Y is a function of independent factor X.

$$Y = F(X) \qquad \text{(Eq. 5.1)}$$

So, the ideal response is obtained by controlling the values of independent variables, i.e. X. Data obtained from various combinations are analyzed to create equations that predict the relationship between cause and effect. For example, the effect of compression time on hardness of tablets is to be ascertained. Hardness obtained at different compression times is to be analyzed statistically. If the correlation coefficient of dissolution time versus hardness is less than 0.5, we assume no relationship exists. But time versus log hardness may result in a correlation coefficient of 0.9. Thus, ruling out the possibility of a direct compression time versus hardness relationship, we would accept compression time versus log of hardness relationship.

If an equation contains only one independent variable, it is assigned different values and responses are measured. The first derivative of the response (dY/dX) shows how the values of response (Y) change with the change of independent factor (X). When there are limiting values like maximum or minimum, setting the value of dY/dX to 0 often gives the solution for X at extreme limits.

If optimization involves more than one variable, statistical design is used and values are analyzed by multiple linear regression analysis.

By carrying out multiple regression analysis, we can determine the influence of a specific factor or interaction of a number of factors on the overall result. Factorial design and simplex method are the two important approaches to achieve this.

Optimization using Factorial Design

Factorial design is nothing but a guideline for experimental plan. For a given number of factors, it gives number of experiments to be carried out as well as quantities of the variable ingredients to be used in the experiments. The basic principle is to change level of one factor keeping the levels of other factors constant. Once the design is framed, products are made according to these formulas. The responses obtained from the products are analyzed for the main and interaction effects. The results are analyzed for the significance of effects too.

Multiple regression analysis (MRA) is carried out to find the relationships between overall response and the different factors. ANOVA is used to find out the errors of the experiments. This helps in finding the confidence level of the evaluated results. Usually, by feeding the response values and the variables in the statistical softwares, an equation (usually a polynomial) is generated. The resulting equation is the basis of optimization and is used as a predictive model. Now, substituting the desired values of response (Y) in the predictive equation, we get the approximate value of independent variables, which are likely to generate the target response. Next, a product is made with the optimized formula, which is validated by actual evaluation.

In factorial designs, the optimization procedure is facilitated by fitting of an empirical polynomial equation to the experimental results. The equation constructed from a 2^n factorial experiment will have 2^n terms.

The generalized expression is,

$$Y = B_0 + B_1X_1 + B_2X_2 + B_3X_3 + B_{12}X_1X_2 + B_{13}X_1X_3 + B_{23}X_2X_3 + B_{123}X_1X_2X_3 \quad \text{(Eq. 5.2)}$$

Here, Y is the measured response and X_i is the level of the ith factor. B_i, B_{ij}, B_{ijk}, etc. represent coefficients of factors and interaction terms computed from the responses of the experimental formulation. From eight formulations, eight responses or eight values of Y are obtained. If the low levels are all zero, all the terms except B_0 become zero.

For example, consider an experiment in which, we would like to assess the effect of three ingredients drug, disintegrant and anti-adherent, concentration on the dissolution time of a tablet (Table 5.1).

Table 5.1: Quantities of ingredients at different levels (Experiment 1)

Factors	*Low level*	*High level*
X_1 = Drug (mg)	0	10
X_2 = Disintegrant (mg)	0	5
X_3 = Anti-adherents (mg)	0	2

Table 5.2: Results of the 2^3 factorial experiments used for construction of the polynomial equation

Formulation code	*Drug (mg)*	*Disintegrant (mg)*	*Anti-adherent (mg)*	*Dissolution time (minutes)*
1	0	0	0	20
X_1	10	0	0	24
X_2	0	5	0	18
X_1X_2	10	5	0	21
X_3	0	0	2	40
X_1X_3	10	0	2	43
X_2X_3	0	5	2	37
$X_1X_2X_3$	10	5	2	39

At low level $X_1 = X_2 = X_3 = 0$.

So, substituting the values of the factors in Eq. 5.2, we get,

$$Y = B_0 + B_1(0) + B_2(0) + B_3(0) + B_{12}(0)(0) + B_{13}(0)(0) + B_{23}(0)(0) + B_{123}(0)(0)(0)$$

$$Y = B_0 = 20 \qquad \text{(Eq. 5.3)}$$

Similarly, the response of the formulation where the first factor is only at the high level and all others are at low level will return the value of coefficient.

When only X_1 is at high level, the response is 24, 18 when X_2 is at high level and 40 when X_3 is at high level. Under such conditions, the value of all interaction terms X_1X_2, X_2X_3, X_1X_3 and $X_1X_2X_3$ are 0.

Substituting the value of B_0 (Eq. 5.3) in the Eq. 5.2, we get the value of B_1, B_2 and B_3.

$$24 = 20 + 10B_1 + B_2(0) + B_3(0) + B_{12}(10)(0) + B_{13}(10)(0) + B_{23}(0)(0) + B_{123}(10)(0)(0).$$

$$24 = 20 + 10B_1 \text{ or } B_1 = 0.4 \qquad \text{(Eq. 5.4)}$$

$$18 = 20 + 5B_2 \text{ or } B_2 = -0.4 \qquad \text{(Eq. 5.5)}$$

$$40 = 20 + 2B_3 \text{ or } B_3 = 10 \qquad \text{(Eq. 5.6)}$$

Similarly, the values of coefficients of the interaction terms B_{12}, B_{13}, B_{23}, B_{123} can be obtained by substituting values of known coefficients.

As X_1X_2 interaction is possible, only when both the ingredients are present in the formulation, to get the value of B_{12}, we should take the response where both X_1 and X_2 are at high level.

The formulation X_1X_2 (response 21) is to be chosen as this meets the condition.

Substituting the values of factors in Eq. 5.2, we get,

$$21 = 20 + 10B_1 + 5B_2 + B_{12}(10)(5)$$

Substituting for the values of B_1 and B_2 from Eq. 5.4 and 5.5.

$$-1 = 50B_{12} \text{ or } B_{12} = -0.02 \qquad \text{(Eq. 5.7)}$$

For B_{13}, we should take the response where both X_1 and X_3 are at high level and X_2 is 0.

Response for this formulation is 43.

So the Eq. 5.2 reduces to:

$$43 = 20 + 10B_1 + B_3(2) + B_{13}(10)(2)$$

Substituting for the values of B_1 and B_3 from Eq. 5.4 and 5.6, we get,

$$-1 = 20B_{13} \text{ or } B_{13} = -0.05 \qquad \text{(Eq. 5.8)}$$

Similarly, for B_{23}, we should take the response where both X_2 and X_3 are at high level and X_1 is 0, the response which fits this condition is 37.

$$37 = 20 + B_2(5) + B_3(2) + B_{23}(5)(2)$$

Putting the values of B_2 and B_3, B_{23} is found to be

$$37 = 20 - 2 + 20 + 10 B_{23}$$

$$B_{23} = -0.1 \quad \text{(Eq. 5.9)}$$

To find the value of B_{123}, the values of all the main and interaction terms are to be substituted and the response to the formulation in which all factors are present in high level should be chosen. This response is 39.

$$39 = B_0 + B_1(10) + B_2(5) + B_3(2) + B_{12}(10)(5) + B_{13}(10)(2) + B_{23}(5)(2) + B_{123}(10)(5)(2)$$

Substituting the values of coefficients and response the equation reduces to

$$39 = 20 + 0.4(10) - 0.4(5) + 10(2) - 0.02(10)(5) - 0.05(10)(2) - 0.1(5)(2) + B_{123}(100)$$

$$39 = 39 + B_{123}(100)$$

$$B_{123} = 0 \quad \text{(Eq. 5.10)}$$

So, the final predictive model is

$$Y = B_0 + 0.4X_1 - 0.4X_2 + 10X_3 - 0.02X_1X_2 - 0.05X_1X_3 - 0.1X_2X_3 \quad \text{(Eq. 5.11)}$$

The term B_{123} has value 0, hence it is omitted from the equation. Some of the terms like X_1X_2, X_1X_3, X_2X_3 have low coefficients. ANOVA is performed to see whether these terms are significant or not (see factorial design chapter). The insignificant terms should be excluded from the final equation.

In short the optimization by factorial design is a sequence of events, which can be summarized as follows.

Decision: → 2^n or 3^n according to the number and level of factors

↓

Choice of high and low level

↓

Formula designing

↓

Production and evaluation (generating response)

↓

Making of a predictive equation

↓

Dropping of insignificant terms (by ANOVA)

↓

Designing of optimized formula on the basis of predictive model

↓

Production and evaluation of the optimized formulation to confirm the validity of the predictive model

Since the lower level of all the factors is zero, in the given example of factorial experiment, the calculation is simple. But in reality lower levels are rarely zero. For example, in tableting, without a certain amount of glidant the powders do not flow from the hopper and a minimum quantity of the binders must be present for binding. Increased amount of binder may give excellent tablets but delay the dissolution time. In such cases, calculation of the effects is more complicated. Suppose, in a 3 factor two level design, X_1 has lower level 2 mg and higher level 6 mg, for X_2 the lower level is 2 and higher level is 8 mg while high and low levels of X_3 are 1 and 10 mg as in Table 5.3.

Table 5.3: Factors and level of a 2^3 factorial experiment (low levels are not zero)

Drug (X_1)	2 (Low)	6 (High)
Disintegrant (X_2)	2 (Low)	8 (High)
Diluent (X_3)	1 (Low)	10 (High)

Developing predictive equations with such actual quantities is difficult as none of the terms will be 0. Designing of formulations can be done with these actual quantities but for the purpose of calculation transformations are needed (Table 5.4).

Table 5.4: Results of the 2^3 factorial experiments used for construction of the polynomial equation

Formulation code	*Drug (X_1) (mg)*	*Disintegrant (X_2) (mg)*	*Diluent (X_3) (mg)*	*Response (minutes)*
1	2	2	1	60
2	6	2	1	45
3	2	8	1	55
4	6	8	1	30
5	2	2	10	58
6	6	2	10	40
7	2	8	10	54
8	6	8	10	20

In the analysis of data obtained from factorial design, once the levels of the factors are transformed, the responses obtained from different experiments are treated with the transformed values to determine the main and interaction effects of different factors. In transformation (often known as coding) all higher values are converted to +1 and lower values to −1.

The formula for the transformation is as follows

$$\frac{\textbf{X} - \textbf{The average of the 2 levels}}{\textbf{1/2 (Differences of the values)}}$$

Let us assume the coded values of X_1, X_2 and X_3 be X_1', X_2' and X_3' respectively.

$$X_1' = \frac{X_1 - 1/2\,(2+6)}{1/2\,(6-2)} = \frac{X_1 - 4}{2} \qquad \text{(Eq. 5.12)}$$

When higher value of X_1, i.e. 6 is fit into this formula, the value becomes

$$\frac{6-4}{2} = 1$$

When the lower level of X_1, i.e. 2 is put into this formula it becomes

$$\frac{2-4}{2} = -1$$

Similarly, X_2' or the coded or transformed formulas for X_2 and X_3 are,

$$X_2' = \frac{X_2 - 1/2\,(2+8)}{1/2\,(8-2)} = \frac{X_2 - 5}{3} \qquad \text{(Eq. 5.13)}$$

$$X_3' = \frac{X_3 - 1/2\,(1+10)}{1/2\,(10-1)} = \frac{X_3 - 5.5}{4.5} \qquad \text{(Eq. 5.14)}$$

A table is constructed in which each column is devoted to one of the possible effects (main and interaction). Table 5.5 contains the transformed values of factors.

Note that the interactions are also represented by +1 or −1. In formulation 1, X_1X_2 is represented by +1 as both X_1 and X_2 have got values of −1 and (−1) × (−1) = 1. But $X_1X_2X_3$ has the value −1 as (−1) (−1) (−1) = −1.

Table 5.5: Transformed levels of factors with signs (used in the determination of effects and polynomial coefficients) X_1', X_2' and X_3'

Code	X_1'	X_2'	X_3'	$X_1'X_2'$	$X_2'X_3'$	$X_1'X_3'$	$X_1'X_2'X_3'$	Total	Response
1	−1	−1	−1	+1	+1	+1	−1	+1	60
2	+1	−1	−1	−1	+1	−1	+1	+1	45
3	−1	+1	−1	−1	−1	+1	+1	+1	55
4	+1	+1	−1	+1	−1	−1	−1	+1	30
5	−1	−1	+1	+1	−1	−1	+1	+1	58
6	+1	−1	+1	−1	−1	+1	−1	+ 1	40
7	−1	+1	+1	−1	+1	−1	−1	+1	54
8	+1	+1	+1	+1	+1	+1	+1	+1	20

The coefficients for a particular factor are calculated using the product of response values multiplied by the sign of that particular column. Each row of the total column of Table 5.5 is assigned the value of +1, which is used to calculate the value of B_0.

To calculate the coefficients for a particular term, e.g. X_1, X_2 or X_1X_2, etc. we have to multiply the response value with the signs and finally add all the values under a particular column-head. Say the coefficient B_1 will be sum total of terms, i.e. response × (−1) or (+1) in the column-head B_1 divided by the total number of formulations. Since all the signs in the total column are positive, all values will be multiplied by +1, then added and averaged to find the value of B_0.

Similarly, the coefficients for X_1, X_2, X_3 and interaction factor (X_1X_2, X_2X_3, X_3X_1 $X_1X_2X_3$) are calculated. In the total column all are positive, i.e. +1. So the total is positive too. The total is divided by 8, which is number of terms in the column (Table 5.6).

Table 5.6: Calculation of coefficients of main and interaction effects

B_0	B_1	B_2	B_3	B_{12}	B_{23}	B_{13}	B_{123}
60	−60	−60	−60	60	60	60	−60
45	45	−45	−45	−45	45	−45	45
55	−55	55	−55	−55	−55	55	55
30	30	30	−30	30	−30	−30	−30
58	−58	−58	58	58	−58	−58	58
40	40	−40	40	−40	−40	40	−40
54	−54	54	54	−54	54	−54	−54
20	20	20	20	20	20	20	20
Adding the columns							
362	−92	−44	−18	−26	−4	−12	−6

Dividing each column total by 8, we get the value of coefficients for a particular term. Therefore, the values obtained for B_0, B_1, B_2, B_3, B_{12}, B_{23}, B_{13}, B_{123} are:

$$B_0 = 362/8 = 45.25.$$
$$B_1 = -92/8 = -11.5.$$
$$B_2 = -44/8 = -5.5.$$
$$B_3 = -18/8 = -2.25.$$
$$B_{12} = -26/8 = -3.25.$$
$$B_{23} = -4/8 = -0.5.$$
$$B_{13} = -12/8 = -1.5.$$
$$B_{123} = -6/8 = -0.75.$$

The coded equation will be

$$Y = 45.25 - 11.5X_1' - 5.5X_2' - 2.25X_3' - 3.25X_1'X_2' - 0.5X_2'X_3' - 1.5X_1'X_3' - 0.75X_1'X_2'X_3' \quad \text{(Eq. 5.15)}$$

The earlier equation (Eq. 5.11) used the untransformed actual values, whereas the present equation (Eq. 5.15) uses coded or transformed values. In transformation, low and high levels are converted to −1 and +1 to allow easy calculation of the coefficients. However, a pertinent question arises whether all the coefficients are significant or not. Each coefficient can be estimated for test of significance by using a *t* test. When coefficient is found to be insignificant, it indicates that the factors or the interactions do not have much influence on the overall response. However, without an estimate of standard deviation, the *t* test cannot be done. Usually, these values (s.d.) are obtained from previous similar experiments. Suppose, for a particular coefficient, s.d. obtained from previous experiments is 1.5 with a d.f. of 16.

From the t table (Appendix 2) we can see that for a two-sided t test with d.f. 16 and 95% confidence level, the value of t is 2.12. The observed t value for coefficient of the term $X_1' X_2' X_3'$ is

$$t = \frac{|0.75|}{1.5/\sqrt{8}} = 1.414$$

Since this value is lesser than 2.12 ($P > 0.05$) the coefficient $X_1' X_2' X_3'$ is not significant. Similarly, t value for the coefficient of $X_2' X_3'$ is 0.94 and $P > 0.05$.

From this we can see that both interaction terms X_{23} and X_{123} are insignificant.

Omitting the insignificant terms the coded equation (Eq. 5.15) reduces to:

$$Y = 45.25 - 11.5X_1' - 5.5X_2' - 2.25X_3' - 3.25X_1'X_2' - 1.5X_1'X_3' \quad \text{(Eq. 5.16)}$$

Suppose, we are interested in getting the response of a formulation where X_1, X_2 and X_3 are 3 mg each. First, the level of ingredients needs to be coded and then the coded values would be substituted in the predictive equation.

The value of X_1' in the coded equation (Eq. 5.15) is $\frac{X_1 - 4}{2}$.

So, if 3 mg is the actual quantity of X_1, the coded value will be

$$\frac{3-4}{2} = -0.5.$$

Similarly, other levels of other factors will be determined and substituted in the equation. To use the actual values in an equation directly, we have to decode the equation.

Decoding the Equation

To get the equation with actual quantities, we have to decode the terms.

As X_1' (the coded value of X_1) is equal to $\frac{X_1 - 4}{2}$, it will be replaced by $\frac{X_1 - 4}{2}$.

Similarly, X_2' and X_3' will be substituted by $\frac{X_2 - 5}{3}$ and $\frac{X_3 - 5.5}{4.5}$.

Substituting these values in the Eq. 5.15 we get,

$$Y = 45.25 - 11.5\left(\frac{X_1 - 4}{2}\right) - 5.5\left(\frac{X_2 - 5}{3}\right) - 2.25\left(\frac{X_3 - 5.5}{4.5}\right)$$

$$- 3.25\left(\frac{X_1 - 4}{2}\right)\left(\frac{X_2 - 5}{3}\right) - 0.5\left(\frac{X_2 - 5}{3}\right)\left(\frac{X_3 - 5.5}{4.5}\right)$$

$$- 1.5\left(\frac{X_1 - 4}{2}\right)\left(\frac{X_3 - 5.5}{4.5}\right) - 0.75\left(\frac{X_2 - 5}{3}\right)\left(\frac{X_1 - 4}{2}\right)\left(\frac{X_3 - 5.5}{4.5}\right)$$

Solving the equation we get,

$$Y = 67.71 - 2.89X_1 - 0.07X_2 - 0.2X_3 - 0.39X_1X_2 - 0.028X_2X_3$$
$$+ 0.074X_1X_3 - 0.028X_1X_2X_3 \quad \text{(Eq. 5.17)}$$

The equation developed in the given example is expected to predict the response within the experimental space of the equations but we must remember that it is just a probability. Without testing some extra design formulations, there is no way to ensure that the empirical equation will be adequate to predict the responses of new formulations. Figure 5.1 shows the experimental spaces within which Eqs 5.11 and 5.17 are supposed to be valid. Usually, to check this point at least one new (not included in design) formulation is made and evaluated and finally compared with the predicted value obtained from the equation.

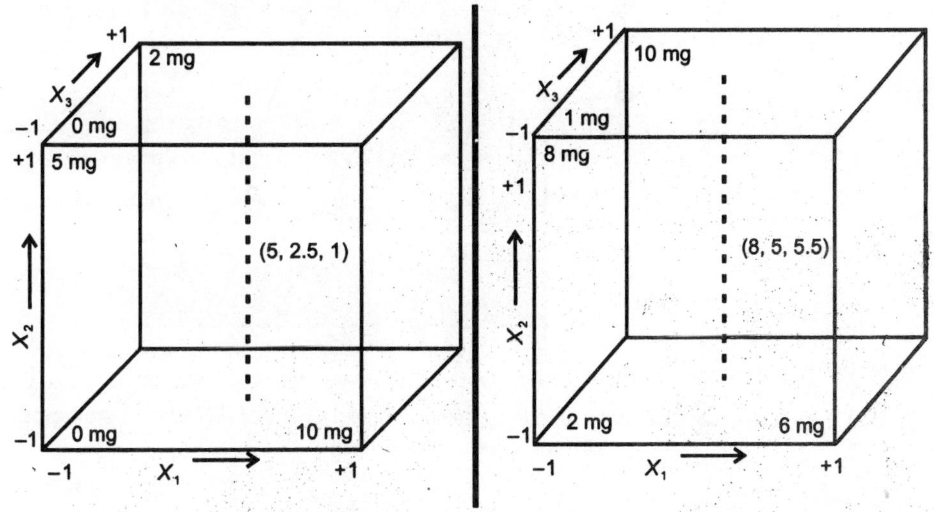

Fig. 5.1: Experimental space described by the Table 5.1 (left) and Table 5.3 (right)

Extrapolation of the predicted value outside the factor space is not desired. Sometimes, predictions are done beyond experimental space too but the probability of getting an accurate response is much lesser than the formulations covered within the factorial space.

Once the predictive equation is verified for its predictive power, optimum formulation can be designed by various methods. Usually, grid method is used to identify the optimum regions and response surface are generated (Table 5.7).

Table 5.7: Grid solutions for responses (Y) based on Eq. 5.16

X_1'	X_2'	X_3'	Y	X_1'	X_2'	X_3'	Y	X_1'	X_2'	X_3'	Y
−1	−1	−1	59.75	0	−1	−1	53.0	1	−1	−1	46.25
−1	−1	0	59.0	0	−1	0	50.75	1	−1	0	42.5
−1	−1	1	58.25	0	−1	1	48.5	1	−1	1	38.75
−1	0	−1	57.5	0	0	−1	47.5	1	0	−1	37.5
−1	0	0	56.75	0	0	0	45.25	1	0	0	33.75
−1	0	1	56.0	0	0	1	43.0	1	0	1	30.0
−1	1	−1	55.25	0	1	−1	42.0	1	1	−1	28.75
−1	1	0	54.5	0	1	0	39.75	1	1	0	25.0
−1	1	1	53.75	0	1	1	37.5	1	1	1	21.25

Indication can also be found from response surface curves

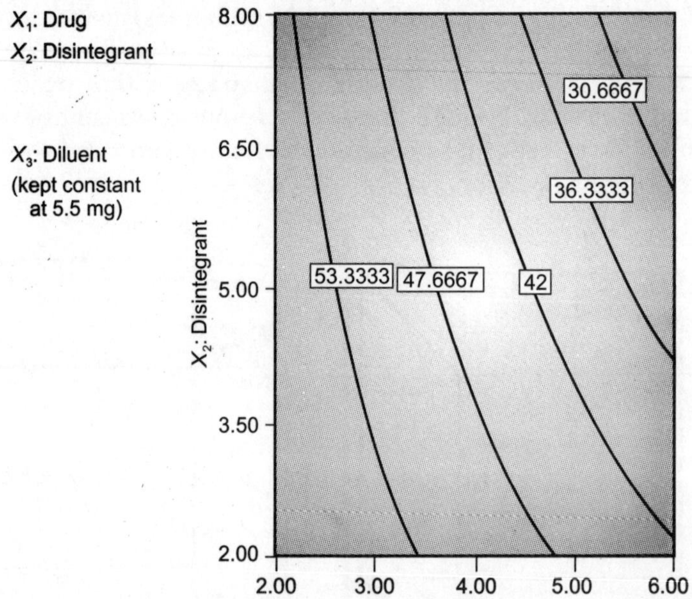

Fig. 5.2: Response surface curve showing the combined effect of drug and disintegrant (diluent is fixed at 5.5 mg)

A response surface shows the response as a function of factor level. If the number of factors are more than two, response surface cannot be presented in a two-dimensional space. In that case, response surface is drawn for two factors only (variable) keeping all the other factors constant.

In the given response surface curve (Fig. 5.2), the response (dissolution time) at varying compositions of drug and disintegrant is shown, while the quantity of diluent is kept constant at the level of 5.5 mg. There are five lines in the figure, which have divided the total space into six sections. Area left to the line marked by 53.33 has values higher than 53.33, i.e. any composition falling in this area will have dissolution time greater than 53.3 minutes. For example, the left lower corner of the figure represents the value $X_1 = 2$, $X_2 = 2$ while X_3 is 5.5 mg (constant for this curve). In coded terms these quantities are represented by –1, –1 and 0. The grid solution for this composition shows a predicted dissolution time of 59 minutes, which is higher than 53.33 minutes.

Similarly, the area enclosed between the lines marked by 53.33 and 47.66 indicates dissolution time between these two values. From these, we can predict the response of a particular combination.

Suppose, we want to find out the composition of a formulation which has dissolution time of 35 minutes, the area between lines marked by 36.3 to 30.6 will provide a set of compositions, the dissolution time of which is likely to be 35 minutes. At any point within this area, the values of X_1 and X_2 can be obtained by cutting perpendicular to the corresponding axis. It saves us from the burden of repeated calculation and allows experimenter to choose the best option for a desired response.

The response surface discussed previously is shown in a three-dimensional form in Fig. 5.3. The surface below is similar to response surface curve shown in Fig. 5.2. The response is shown in the upper surface. The upper surface hangs like a slanted roof above the lower surface which shows the composition of drug and disintegrant.

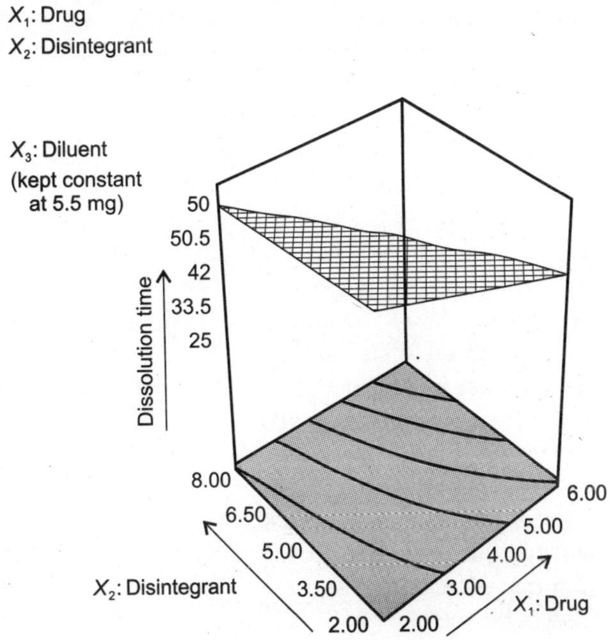

Fig. 5.3: Three-dimensional representation of response at fixed diluent concentration (dissolution time is shown at various composition of drug and disintegrant)

It is apparent that the highest elevation of the upper curve is just above intersecting point of 2.0 and 2.0 and the lowest depression is just opposite to this point. Grid solution shows the highest dissolution time when diluent is kept at 0 level (5.5 mg) coincides with −1, −1 (2 mg of drug and 2 mg of disintegrant) and the value is 59 minutes. However, reading a three-dimensional curve is more difficult than two-dimensional response surface curves. Suppose, we are interested in a dissolution time of 35 minutes. We have to find the value 35 in the dissolution scale first. From this point, we have to imagine a line drawn parallel to X_1 axis that appears to cut the slanting upper surface at a particular point. The corresponding point on the lower surface would give the composition of the formulation that has dissolution time of 35 minutes.

Simplex Lattice

A simplex is a geometric figure that has one more point than the number of factors. For example, if two independent variables are involved, simplex will be a triangle. This class of design is useful for optimization procedure where the total quantity of ingredients is constant. Suppose, syrup is being designed. Here, it is already decided that 80% is solvent and other ingredients like viscosity inducers, coloring agent and sweeteners comprise 20% of the weight. If we want to investigate the effect of these ingredients on the overall quality of syrup, the concentration of these factors would be varied in a systematic manner with the restriction that the total concentration of the solute is always 80%.

To clarify the concept, let us take a simple example. Suppose, the drug is poorly soluble and we would like to use a combination solvent in which the drug has good solubility.

To begin with, combination of solvents are taken in such a way that the experimental data will be able to predict the responses, i.e. solubility of drug over the entire simplex space. The simplex space is the space enclosed by the various combinations of solvents chosen for the experiment.

A very simple diagram is shown in Fig. 5.4. Here, A and B are 2 solvents which are used in combination to dissolve the drug. The aim of the experiment is to choose the solvent system in which the drug has maximum solubility. Since, no other solvent is allowed apart from A and B, the restriction of this system is that the total quantity of A and B should always be 100%.

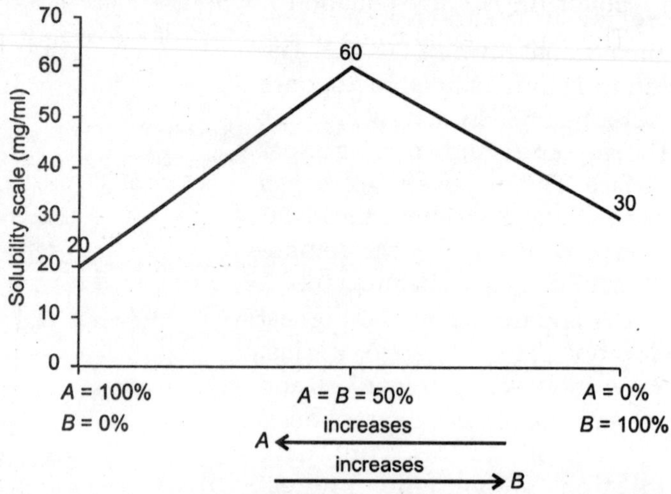

Fig. 5.4: Two-component solvent system used to illustrate the simplex approach of optimization

The simplest design suggests a minimum of 3 experiments.

(*a*) Determination of solubility of the drug in 100% A

(*b*) Determination of solubility of the drug in 100% B

(*c*) Determination of solubility of the drug in a mixture of 50% A and 50% B.

The symbol Y represents the response (solubility of drug in these 3 systems).

Let B_1, B_2 and B_{12} be the symbols representing the results of the experiments while the experimental values of solubility are 20, 30 and 60 mg/ml respectively. Using this system we have to develop an equation, which will show the overall solubility (Y) as a function of proportion or fraction of individual solvents.

The overall solubility of drug in the mixture can result from the main effect of A, main effect of B and interaction effects of A and B. In pure A or B, it can only be due to the main effect of A or B whereas the mixture of A and B can have an interaction effect too. Hence, the generalized equation that takes into consideration every possibility is,

$$Y = B_1(A) + B_2(B) + B_{12}(A)(B) \qquad \text{(Eq. 5.18)}$$

This indicates the overall solubility in a mixture can result from the main effect of A, main effect of B and interaction effects of A and B.

In this equation, the proportion of each component is indicated by decimal rather than %. Here, 1 represents 100%, i.e. the concentration of pure A or B. Similarly, 50% is 0.5 and 25% is 0.25.

To calculate the coefficients of A and B, we have to substitute the experimental results of pure A and B in Eq. 5.18.

As $A + B = 1$ when A is 1 the value of B is 0.
For 100% A ..... $(A) = 1$ and $(B) = 0$
So for 100% A, the equation $Y = B_1(1) + B_2(0) + B_{12}(1)(0)$ reduces to $Y = B_1(1)$.
The experimental value of solubility of the drug in pure A is 20 mg/ml.

$$B_1 = 20 \qquad \text{(Eq. 5.19)}$$

Similarly, for 100% B, $(B) = 1$. So $(A) = 0$.
The equation reduces to $Y = B_2(1)$.

$$B_2 = 30 \qquad \text{(Eq. 5.20)}$$

The values of B_1 and B_2 are used for calculating the value of B_{12} in Eq. (5.18).

$$Y = B_1(A) + B_2(B) + B_{12}(A)(B)$$
$$60 = 20\,(0.5) + 30\,(0.5) + B_{12}(0.5)\,(0.5)$$
$$B_{12}(0.25) = 60 - 25$$
$$B_{12} = 35/0.25$$
$$B_{12} = 140 \qquad \text{(Eq. 5.21)}$$

By substituting the values of B_1, B_2 and B_{12}, the final equation is found to be,

$$Y = 20\,(A) + 30\,(B) + 140\,(A)\,(B) \qquad \text{(Eq. 5.22)}$$

The value of B_{12} can be derived from a logical reasoning too. The formula to obtain B_{12} by this reasoning is given by,

$$B_{12} = 4\,(\text{Solubility at 50–50 mixture of } A \text{ and } B)$$
$$-\,2\,(\text{Sum of solubility at } A = 1 \text{ and } B = 1)$$

The logic is simple. In 1 ml of 50 – 50 mixture of A and B, we have got 0.5 ml A and 0.5 ml B. Multiplied by 4, it makes 4 ml in which 2 ml should be A and rest 2 ml B. If there is no interaction between A and B, the total solubility of any moiety in this system should be equal to the solubility in 2 ml of A and 2 ml of B.

The first term at the right hand side of the expression represents solubility of the drug in 4 parts of 50–50 mixture of A and B whereas the second term indicates the sum of solubility in 2 parts of pure A and 2 parts of pure B. If both the terms are not equal it indicates an interaction.

In the absence of interaction both the values, i.e. 4 (Solubility at 50 – 50 mixture of A and B) and 2 (Sum of solubility at $A = 1$ and $B = 1$) are equal and the value of B_{12} is 0.

A positive value of B_{12} indicates that there is some interaction between A and B, which gives positive effect or enhances solubility. Negative value indicates there is antagonism or the interaction between A and B reduces solubility.

The response equation can predict responses at extra design points. We can have results for percentage combinations of solvents for which no experiment is conducted. Of the three experimental values, the highest value was obtained from the 50 – 50 mixture of A and B. However, it does not necessarily indicate that this combination has the highest solubility. To get a comprehensive picture of the solubility profile, we have to perform experiments at some extra design combinations and validate these from the predictive equation.

But if we use another solvent C where total of $A + B + C = 1$, this equation is not valid because $A + B = 1$ is the constraint of the equation.

Figure 5.4 shows as the graph moves from left to right, the percentage of A decreases and percentage of B increases. Here, B_1, B_2 and B_{12} are the results of the experiment and the values are 20, 30 and 60 mg/ml respectively. Once a diagram is drawn, we can find the solubility at other points by drawing a vertical line to the curve from X-axis. The value of Y at the point of interaction will show the solubility. Correspondingly, for a desired solubility, we have to draw perpendicular line from the curve to the X-axis.

Equation 5.22 can also predict the maximum solubility. It is calculated by setting the first derivative as 0. It is assumed, at the peak (where the solubility is maximum), even if the composition of solvent changes the solubility does not. So dY, i.e. change in response (solubility) with respect to a small change in the proportion of A or B (dA or dB) is 0.

$$Y = 20\,(A) + 30\,(B) + 140\,(A)\,(B) \qquad \text{(Eq. 5.22)}$$

Since $A + B = 1$, B is $1 - A$.

$$Y = 20\,(A) + 30\,(1 - A) + 140\,(A)\,(1 - A)$$
$$Y = 20\,(A) + 30 - 30A + 140A - 140A^2$$

The first derivative of the equation is dY/dA.

When $dY/dA = 0$, Eq. 5.22 reduces to,

$$dY/dA = 20 + 0 - 30 + 140 - 280A$$
$$0 = 130 - 280A$$
$$A = 130/280$$
$$A = 0.46$$

It indicates when fraction of A is 0.46 or 46%, the highest solubility will be attained.

In general, simplex design is used to solve formulation problems when the effect of 3 or more components is evaluated on the overall response.

The design is represented by regular sided figures, like triangular or rectangular with all sides equal or pentagonal with all arms equal. With more than 4 components in a single formula, figures cannot be easily constructed but it can be expressed by the theoretical thought of an N-sided figure in the $N - 1$ dimension space.

If we have 3 components in a formulation, we will have 7 experiments; 3 with pure ingredients like 100% A, 100% B and 100% C. There will also be 4 possible interaction effects. So we have to perform a minimum of 7 experiments.

Similarly, for a 4-component mixture of A, B, C, D, we have four main effects (100% A, 100% B, 100% C and 100% D), 6 second (low order) interaction (AB, BC, CD, BD, AC, AD), 4 third order interaction (ABC, BCD, ABD, ACD) and one fourth order interaction ($ABCD$).

To assess second order interactions, the proportions of A and B are equal (50% of both). For third order interaction, the proportions of A, B and C in the mixture are 33% of each ingredient. For fourth order interaction, the proportion of each ingredient would be 25%.

For three-component system the generalized polynomial equation will be,

$$Y = B_a(A) + B_b(B) + B_c(C) + B_{ab}(A)(B) + B_{ac}(A)(C) + B_{bc}(B)(C) + B_{abc}(A)(B)(C) \quad \text{(Eq. 5.23)}$$

For four-component system it would be

$$Y = B_a(A) + B_b(B) + B_c(C) + B_d(D) + B_{ab}(A)(B) + B_{ac}(A)(C) + B_{bc}(B)(C) + \ldots + B_{abc}(A)(B)(C) + B_{bcd}(B)(C)(D) + \ldots + B_{abcd}(A)(B)(C)(D) \quad \text{(Eq. 5.24)}$$

When $A = 1$ all other terms become zero

$$Y = B_a(A)$$

$$Y = B_a(1)$$

$$Y = B_a$$

Similarly, when B and C take the value of 1, B_b, B_c is determined.

$$Y = B_b$$

$$Y = B_c$$

Once the value of B_a and B_b are known, the coefficient of the higher order interaction like B_{ab} can be determined. Similarly, once the lower order interaction is known, their values can be substituted to find out higher order interactions.

Sequential Optimization

Let us think of a situation, where it is desired to have a specific dissolution time of 15 minutes of a tablet by adjusting 3 variables; disintegrant, lubricant and fill weight. In n factor factorial experiment, where each factor is studied at 2 levels, total number of experiments will be 2^n or 8. Moreover, the eight experiments will not be able to predict the response equation accurately, if any of the factors has non-linear response profile. Sequential optimization starts with much lesser number of initial experiments. In n factor experiment, total number of initial experiments is $n + 1$. Since we have 3 factors, $n = 3$, number of initial experiments will be $n + 1$, i.e. 4. The first problem is the designing of initial formulae. Like factorial experiments, the high (+) and low levels (–) of each factor need to be fixed. Usually, the initial $n + 1$ formulations are designed by keeping each of the factors at high level once, while other factors are at low level.

Let us code the disintegrant as A, lubricant as B and fill weight as C. Hence for the first 3 initial formulations, A, B and C each is used at high level (+), while others are at low level (–). In the last, i.e. $(n + 1)$th experiment, all the factors are taken at high level (+ + +).

Let us assume,

For A, low and high levels are 0 and 50 mg.

For B, low and high levels are 0.2 and 2 mg.

For C, low and high levels are 100 and 250 mg.

The target dissolution is 15 minutes.

Table 5.8: Formula for initial four experiments for a three factor sequential simplex

Formulation	*Disintegrant (A) (mg)*		*Lubricant (B) (mg)*		*Fill weight (C) (mg)*		*Response (minutes)*
Code	*Level*	*Quantity*	*Level*	*Quantity*	*Level*	*Quantity*	
I_1	+	50	–	0.2	–	100	17
I_2	–	0	+	2.0	–	100	38
I_3	–	0	–	0.2	+	250	26
I_4	+	50	+	2.0	+	250	20

Here I_1, I_2 and I_3 each has one factor at high level and I_4 the last experiment has all the factors at high level. Once the formulations are made and evaluated, the responses should be compared with the target response. Table 5.8 shows that none of the responses meets the target of 15 minutes.

To continue the optimization procedure, new formulations are designed. The new formulations are designed according to a sequence. The responses of the initial formulations are ranked according to their closeness to the target response. Since $n + 1$ formulations are there, formulations will have 1, 2...n, $n + 1$ ranks.

As there are 4 formulations, there will be 4 ranks for the initial formulations.

New formulations are made based on the response of the initial formulations. The formula for the new formulations is derived from the existing ones.

Table 5.9: Ranks of initial formulation according to target response

Ranking	*Formulation code*	*Response*
1	I_1	17
2	I_4	20
3	I_3	26
4	I_2	38

The rules for designing the first derived formulation:

Formulation having rank $n + 1$, i.e. the one farthest from the target, is designated as the worst.

First, the quantities of the ingredients used in formulation having the rank 1 to n are averaged to find a formula designated as P.

Next, the quantities of the ingredients in the worst formulation are subtracted from P to get the value of $(P - W)$.

The first derived formulation will have the formula $P + (P - W)$.

Let us assume the code for the first (new) formulation is D_1 as it is derived from existing formulations. Once the response of this new formulation is obtained, it is compared with the response of the first $n + 1$ formulation and also ranked according to the closeness to the target response. Based on the ranking of this D_1 formulation, another new formulation, i.e. D_2 is designed according to a given set of rules.

In Table 5.9, I_2 has the 4th, i.e. $(n + 1)$th rank according to the response. So it is termed as the worst response.

The average term P, for first derived formulation will be calculated from the I_1, I_3 and I_4 and for calculation of $(P - W)$, I_2 will be used.

General guidelines for designing new formulation:

Total number of formulations compared at a given time is $n + 2$ (number of retained formulations is $n + 1$ and 1 derived formulation).

If the new formulation gets the 1st rank, we go to rule no. 1.

Getting rank 1 means its response is better than all the existing formulations or it is better than the best. The formula for the worst formulation is used for calculating the derived formulation in each case.

The formula for rule no. 1 is: $P + 2 (P - W)$.

If a new formulation gets a rank anywhere between 2 to n, we go to rule no 2. The formula for rule no. 2 is: $P + (P - W)$.

Getting a rank of 2 to n indicates that the response is worse than the best but better than the 2nd worst, (i.e. $n + 1$)th response. The new formulation will get the nth rank if its response is better or equal to the previous 2nd worst response.

If the new formulation gets ($n + 1$)th, we go to rule no 3.

The formula for rule no. 3 is: $P + 0.5 (P - W)$.

If the ranking for the new formulation is ($n + 2$)th, we go to rule no. 4.

The formula for rule 4 is: $P - 0.5 (P - W)$.

Suppose, the response of the new formulation is 24. So, according to the response the D_1 gets the 3rd, i.e. the nth rank. The second new formulation D_2 will be designed according to rule no. 2.

If the response of D_2 is 40 minutes, i.e. worse than previous worst, the next new formulation would be designed according to rule no. 4. Sometimes, the new derived formulations have negative quantities, which are impossible to prepare. In such cases also, they are given to the worst rank that is ($n + 2$)th rank and rule 4 is followed.

The values for the impossible formulations are not discarded though actual production is not done. Those formulae are used for calculation of $(P - W)$. In general, once the value of the worst formulation is used in the calculation of $(P - W)$, it is thrown out of the sequence. For comparison purpose, at a given time we have only $n + 2$ formulations, $n + 1$ from the earlier sequence and 1 new (derived) formulation. This sequence is carried until optimal or repeated responses start appearing.

A worked out example illustrating the sequential manner of formulation design.

A fast dissolving tablet is being designed and optimization is to be done with respect to 3 factors—drug (A), disintegrant (B) and fill weight (C). Target disintegration time (DT) is 10 seconds. The low and high levels of A, B, C, chosen for the initial formulations are (0–25), (0.5–2.0) and (100–200) mg respectively. As number of factors is 3, number of initial formulations is 4 (Table 5.10).

Table 5.10: Formula and response of initial formulations (sequential simplex)

Formulation code	*Drug (A) (mg)*	*Disintegrant (B) (mg)*	*Fill wt (C) (mg)*	*Response (DT) (Sec)*
I_1	25	0.5	100	100
I_2	0.0	2.0	100	50
I_3	0.0	0.5	200	80
I_4	25	2.0	200	70

Table 5.11: Ranking of the initial formulations according to target response

Ranking	*Formulation code*	*Response*
1	I_2	50
2	I_4	70
3	I_3	80
4	I_1	100

As target is 10 second, formulation I_1 is the worst. Hence, it is excluded and P is calculated with I_2, I_3 and I_4.

$$I_1 = \text{worst}$$

For A (drug) the average value of the retained formulations is:

$$\frac{0+0+25}{3} = \frac{25}{3} = 8.3 \text{ mg.}$$

For B (disintegrant) the average value of the retained formulation is:

$$\frac{2+0.5+2}{3} = \frac{4.5}{3} = 1.5 \text{ mg.}$$

For C (fill weight) the average value of the retained formulations is:

$$\frac{100+200+200}{3} = \frac{500}{3} = 166.7 \text{ mg.}$$

So, $P = (8.3, 1.5, 166.7)$

Formula for I_1—the worst formulation has quantities 25, 0.5, 100 mg for A, B and C respectively.

$$P - W = (8.3-25), (1.5-0.5), (166.7-100)$$
$$= (-16.7, 1, 66.7) \text{ mg.}$$

The first derived formulation D_1 is to be designed according to the formula $P + (P - W)$.

$$D_1 = (8.3 - 16.7), (1.5 + 1), (166.7 + 66.7)$$
$$= (-8.4, 2.5, 233.4) \text{ mg.}$$

Here, production of D_1 is impossible as the quantity of A is negative. So, it gets the rank $(n + 2)$th, i.e. 5th rank. Hence, once again, P is calculated with I_2, I_3 and I_4. The previous worst I_1 is removed from the formulation series and the ranking of the sequence is changed (Table 5.12).

Table 5.12: Sequence of formulations including the first derived formula

Formulation code	*Drug (A) (mg)*	*Disintegrant (B) (mg)*	*Fill wt (C) (mg)*	*Response (DT) (sec)*
I_2	0	2.0	100	50
I_4	25	2.0	200	70
I_3	0	0.5	200	80
D_1	–8.4	2.5	233.4	–

Here, D_1 is the new worst. So, instead of I_1, which was the worst in the previous sequence, the formula of D_1 is used in calculation of $P - W$. As D_1, the new formulation has ranked last, D_2, the second derived formulation is designed according to rule no. 4.

$$\begin{aligned} D_2 &= (8.3, 1.5, 166.7) - 0.5\,\{[8.3 - (-8.4)], (1.5 - 2.5), (166.7 - 233.4)\} \\ &= (8.3, 1.5, 166.7) - 0.5\,(16.7, -1, -66.7) \\ &= (8.3, 1.5, 166.7) - (8.3, -0.5, -33.3) \\ &= (0.0, 2.0, 200) \end{aligned}$$

The formula for D_2 has real quantities for each factor. Hence, formulation is possible. So, it is formulated and evaluated and ranked for responses (Tables 5.13, 5.14).

Table 5.13: Sequence of formulations with the second derived formula

Formulation code	*Drug (A) (mg)*	*Disintegrant (B) (mg)*	*Fill wt (C) (mg)*	*Response (DT) (sec)*
I_2	0.0	2.0	100	50
I_3	0.0	0.5	200	80
I_4	25	2.0	200	70
D_2	0.0	2.0	200	75

Table 5.14: Ranks of formulations with second derived formula

Ranking	*Formulation code*	*Response*
1	I_2	50
2	I_4	70
3	D_2	75
4	I_3	80

Next P is calculated with I_2, D_2, I_4 and I_3 but instead of D_1 which was the worst in the previous sequence, I_3 is the new worst. D_1, the old worst is thrown out of the sequence. Since D_2 has the nth rank, the new formulation D_3 is designed according to rule no 2. D_3 is to be designed according to the formula $P + (P - W)$.

The new P has the following quantities,

$$\frac{0 + 0 + 25}{3} = \frac{25}{3} = 8.3 \text{ mg for } A.$$

$$\frac{2 + 2 + 2}{3} = 2 \text{ mg for } B.$$

$$\frac{100 + 200 + 200}{3} = \frac{500}{3} = 166.7 \text{ mg for } C.$$

I_3 is the new worst. So, $(P - W) = (8.3 - 0), (2.0 - 0.5), (166.7 - 200)$ mg for A, B and C respectively. So, D_3 is designed as per rule no. 2, i.e. $P + (P - W)$.

Hence, $D_3 = 16.6, 3.5, 133.4$ for A, B, C.

If its response is 76 seconds, it gets 4th or $(n + 1)$th rank.

D_4 is to be designed as per rule no. 3. The formula of D_3 would be the new worst (Table 5.15).

Table 5.15: Sequence of formulations with the third derived formula

Formulation code	*Drug (A) (mg)*	*Disintegrant (B) (mg)*	*Fill wt (C) (mg)*	*Response (DT) (sec)*
I_2	0	2.0	100	50
I_4	25	2.0	200	70
D_2	8.3	2.0	200	75
D_3	16.6	3.5	133.4	76

For A, B and C, $P = 11.1, 2.0, 166.7$ and $P - W$ is $-5.5, -1.5, 33.3$ respectively.

The new formula D_4 has real quantities 8.3, 1.25 and 183.4 for A, B and C respectively and can be formulated and ranked. Let us assume its response to be 30 seconds (Table 5.16).

Table 5.16: Ranking of formulations with the fourth derived formula

Formulation code	*Drug (A) (mg)*	*Disintegrant (B) (mg)*	*Fill wt (C) (mg)*	*Response (DT) (sec)*
D_4	8.3	1.25	183.4	30
I_2	0.0	2.0	100	50
I_4	25	2.0	200	70
D_2	8.3	2.0	200	75

P is calculated with D_4, I_2, I_4 and D_2 is the new worst.

Since D_4 has the ranking of 1, D_5 will be designed as per rule no. 1.

This process is repeated until the optimum response is obtained.

BIBLIOGRAPHY

1. Box, GE, Hunter WG and Hunter JS, statistics for experimenters, John Wiley and Sons, 1978.
2. Davies OL, The design and analysis of industrial experiments, Hafner New York, 1963.
3. De, Muth James E, Basic statistics and pharmaceutical statistical applications, Marcel Dekker, Inc, 1999.
4. Sanford Bolton, *Practical and Clinical Applications*, Third edition, Marcel Dekker, Inc, 1997.

6 Quantitative Structure–Activity Relationship

INTRODUCTION

Quantitative structure–activity relationship (*QSAR*) is the process by which chemical structure is quantitatively correlated with a well-defined process, such as biological activity or chemical reactivity.

For example, biological activity can be expressed quantitatively as a concentration of a compound required to exert a certain biological response. In addition to this, when physiochemical properties or various structure parameters/descriptors of the compounds under investigation are expressed by numbers, one can form a mathematical relationship (or quantitative structure-activity relationship) between the biological activity and the physicochemical property. The mathematical expression generated can then be used to predict the biological response of other chemical structures designed by the scientists for similar activity.

A general mathematical form of QSAR is:

Activity = *f* (physiochemical properties and/or structural properties).

Such types of equations give a formula to relate biological activity to molecular descriptors. Equations of this type are valuable since they allow prediction of activity without actually requiring synthesis and testing of a compound. Molecules that are predicted to have low activity may be avoided, and research can be focused on compounds with a high probability of showing good activity. In practice, to generate a QSAR model, a number of compounds must first be prepared. This series of compounds should have different substituents with a range of properties (electron-donating/withdrawing and lipo/hydrophilic) and measurable biological activity like EC_{50}, IC_{50}, plasma protein binding, receptor affinity, etc. A relationship can be developed using linear regression analysis to find a best-fit line for the data. The regressions, normally performed by either a spreadsheet like Excel or specialized QSAR software, attempt to fit the selected parameters to the experimental biological activity. The results of the regression will be in form of coefficients for the parameters, which have been found to be significant, and an *r*-value for the line. If the parameters are of similar magnitude, the coefficients give an idea of the relative importance of each parameter. A larger coefficient normally indicates a greater dependence on the variable and its related molecular property. The *r*-value relates the goodness of the fit of the line.

Basic Concept

Computational chemistry represents molecular structures as numerical models and simulates their behavior with the equations of quantum and classical physics. Many programs are available, which enable scientists to easily generate and represent a molecule as molecular data including geometries, energies and associated properties (electronic, spectroscopic and bulk). A QSAR attempts to find relationships between the variations in the values of molecular properties and the biological activity for a series of compounds, so that these 'rules' can be used to evaluate new chemical entities.

A QSAR generally takes the form of a linear equation

$$\text{Biological activity} = \text{Const} + (X_1 * P_1) + (X_2 * P_2) + (X_3 * P_3) + \ldots \quad \text{(Eq. 6.1)}$$

where the parameters P_1 through P_n are computed for each molecule in the series and the coefficients X_1 through X_n are calculated by fitting variations in the parameters and the biological activity.

To generate a good QSAR equation it is essential that, the data that we are collecting or generating must fulfill the following objectives:

- Biological activity/drug-receptor binding data should have been measured with sufficient precision and the data should have both the negative and positive values;
- A set of parameters which can be easily obtained and which are likely to be related to receptor affinity;
- A method/software for establishing a relationship between the parameters and activity (the QSAR) and a method for validating the QSAR model.

Usually, a QSAR equation is a linear model, which relates variations in biological activity to variations in the values of computed (or measured) properties for a series of molecules. For the method to work efficiently the compounds selected must be divided into a training set and a test set. The training set compounds will describe the 'chemical space' (i.e. the chemical structures/entities required or not required for the particular activity) of the experiments and should be diverse.

The quality of any QSAR will only be as good as the quality of the input data, which is used to derive the model. Dose-response curves need to be smooth, contain enough points to assure accuracy and should span two or more orders of magnitude. Multiple readings for a given observation should be reproducible and have relatively smaller errors (signal-to-noise ratio). The variation of the readings obtained by repeatedly testing the same compound should be much smaller than the variation over the series. In cases where the data collected from biological experiments do not follow these guidelines, other methods of data analysis should be utilized since the QSAR models derived from the data will be questionable.

Once biological data have been collected, these should not be directly submitted to QSAR analysis. As the biological data are generally found to be skewed, the log transformation moves the data to a nearly normal distribution. Thus, when measuring responses under equilibrium conditions, the most frequent transformation used is to express concentration values (such as IC_{50}, EC_{50}, etc.) as log (C) or log $1/(C)$.

Since the purpose of a QSAR is to highlight relationships between activity and structural features, we would like to find one or more structural features that relate these molecules and their associated activity. Additionally, we would like to find a parameter that works consistently for all of the molecules in the series.

There are several potential classes of parameters used in QSAR studies. Substituent constants and other physicochemical parameters (such as Hammett sigma constants) measure the electronic effects of a group on the molecule. Fragment counts are used to enumerate the presence of specific substructures. Other parameters can include topological descriptors and values derived from quantum chemical calculations.

The first step in any QSAR study is the selection of relevant parameters/descriptors. If the association between the parameter(s) selected and activity is strong, activity predictions will be possible. If there is only weak association, the QSAR equation cannot be used for predicting the activity. Thus, for a given study, parameters should be selected which are relevant to the activity for the series of molecules under investigation and these parameters should have values which are obtained in a consistent manner.

Once a mathematical model has been generated, the first question that comes to mind is—How much confidence should we place in this model? To find out an answer to this question first of all determine how well the equation predicts activities for known compounds in the series. The difference between the calculated values and the actual (or measured) values for each compound is termed the residual from the model. The residuals are one way to quantify the error in the estimate for individual values calculated by the regression equation for this data set. The standard error for the residuals is calculated by taking the root-mean-square of the residuals.

In order to be an improved model, the standard deviation of the residuals calculated from the model should be smaller than the standard deviation of the original data.

There are *several assumptions* inherent in deriving a QSAR model for a series of compounds.

- The calculations/measurement of parameters can be done more accurately and cheaply than activity.
- The deviations from the best-fit line follow a normal (Gaussian) distribution.
- Any variation in the line described by the QSAR equation is independent of the magnitude of both the activity and the parameters.

Variation in the data is quantified by the correlation coefficient, r, which measures how closely the observed data follow the fitted regression line. Errors in either the model or in the data will lead to a bad fit. This indicator of fit to the regression line is calculated as:

$$r^2 = \frac{\text{Sum of squares of deviations from the regression line}}{\text{Sum of squares of the deviations from the mean}}$$

$$r^2 = \frac{\text{Regression variance}}{\text{Original variance}} \qquad \text{(Eq. 6.2)}$$

where the regression variance is defined as the original variance minus the variance around the regression line. The original variance is the sum-of-the-squares distances of the original data from the mean.

Possible values reported for r^2 fall between 0 and 1. An r^2 of 0 means that there is no relationship between activity and the parameter(s) selected for the study. An r^2 of 1 means there is perfect correlation. While the fit of the data to the regression line is excellent, how can one decide if this correlation is based purely on chance? The higher the value for r^2, the less likely that the relationship is due to chance. If many variables are used in a regression equation, it is possible to get a good fit to the data due to the flexibility of the fitting process; a line will fit two points perfectly, a quadratic curve will fit three, multiple linear regression will fit the observed data if there are enough explanatory variables. Given the assumption that the datum has a Gaussian distribution, the F statistic given below assesses the statistical significance of the regression equation.

The F statistic is calculated from r^2 and the number of data points (or degrees of freedom) in the data set. The F ratio is calculated as:

$$F_{m,n} = (n - m - 1)\frac{r^2}{1 - r^2} \qquad \text{(Eq. 6.3)}$$

where n is the number of data set point, m is the number of variables in the final equation, $n - m - 1$ is the degree of freedom. This value often appears as standard output from statistical programs or it can be checked in statistical tables to determine the significance of the regression equation.

Multiple linear regression (MLR): As discussed previously in Chapter 3, conceptually MLR is used to determine the relative importance of multiple variables to the overall fit of the data. It attempts to maximize the fit of the data to a regression equation (minimize the squared deviations from the regression equation) for the biological activity (maximize the r^2 value) by adjusting each of the available parameters up or down. Successive regression equations are derived in stepwise manner, in which parameters are either added or removed until the r^2 and s values are optimized. The magnitude of the coefficients derived in this manner indicates the relative contribution of the associated parameter to biological activity. There are two important forewarnings in applying multiple regression analysis. The first is based on the fact that, if we add enough parameters into the study any data set can be fitted to a regression line. To overcome this problem, a regression analysis generally requires significantly more compounds than parameters; a useful rule of thumb is six times more compounds should be taken into the study as compared to the number of parameters under consideration. The second difficulty is that, the regression analysis is most effective for interpolation (the region of experimental space) and it is the extrapolation (projecting to a new, unanalyzed region) in which a researcher is more interested in, i.e. for the prediction of activity for newly designed compounds. As more terms are added to multiple linear regression, r^2 always gets larger.

Several reviews on QSAR discussing the various aspects of the MLR methods have been reported.

Evolution of QSAR

More than a century ago, Crum-Brown and Fraser expressed the idea that the physiological action of a substance was a function of its chemical composition and constitution. A few decades later, in 1893, Richet showed that the cytotoxicities of a diverse set of simple organic molecules were inversely related to their corresponding water solubilities. At the beginning of the 20th century, Meyer and Overton independently suggested that the narcotic (depressant) action of a group of organic compounds paralleled their olive oil/water partition coefficients. Ferguson, in 1939, introduced a thermodynamic generalization to the correlation of depressant action with the relative saturation of volatile compounds in the vehicle in which they were administered. The extensive work of Albert, Bell and Roblin established the importance of ionization of bases and weak acids in bacteriostatic activity.

Meanwhile on the physical organic front, huge success was made by correlating the effect of substituent on compound's property. This pioneering work was led by Hammett, who gave rise to the (σ, ρ) culture. The electronic parameter, σ, developed by him in his first study, related the electronic effect of a substituent to the difference between log K_a of the substituted and unsubstituted benzoic acids (Eqs 6.4 and 6.5). By definition, the σ value of hydrogen is 0. Since the logarithm of an equilibrium constant is proportional to the free energy change of the reaction (ΔG), σ values measure the free energy change caused by a particular substituent (Eq. 6.6) (Fig. 6.1).

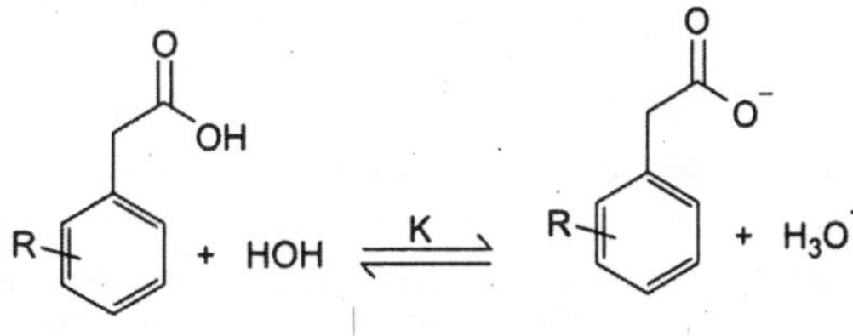

Fig. 6.1: Ionization of a substituted benzoic acid

$$K_a = K\,(H_2O) = \frac{(A^-)(H_3O^+)}{(HA)} \quad \text{(Eq. 6.4)}$$

$$\sigma_R = \log K_{a\,(R)} - \log K_{a\,(H)} \quad \text{(Eq. 6.5)}$$

$$\Delta G = -2.303\ RT \log K \quad \text{(Eq. 6.6)}$$

Taft devised a way for separating polar, steric, and resonance effects and introducing the first steric parameter, ES. The contributions of Hammett and Taft together laid the mechanistic basis for the development of the QSAR paradigm by Hansch and Fujita.

Hansch analysis: A multiple linear regression analysis

In the early 1960s, Corwin Hansch extended the concept of linear-free energy relationships (LFER) to describe the effectiveness of a biologically active molecule. This effort quantitatively related the structure of a compound to its activity, and the resulting equations were aptly named quantitative structure-activity relationships (QSAR). In place of activity if we use any other parameter like lipophilicity, electronic, pharmacokinetic profiles, etc. then these equations are called quantitative structure-property relationships (QSPR). The parameters used to measure electronic properties 'σ' and lipophilicity constant 'π' were developed by Hammett and Hansch respectively.

Many other parameters have been investigated in QSAR equations, but none have found the wide acceptance of σ and π. With these two parameters, a typical QSAR equation takes the form of Eq. 6.7. Note that the π term is present as both π and π^2 since lipophilicity tends to follow a parabolic relationship relative to activity. Log 1/C is a term representing the concentration of a drug needed to achieve a desired level of effect. *k*, *k'*, π, and *k''* are all regression coefficients.

$$\log (1/C) = -k\pi + k'\pi^2 + \rho\sigma + k'' \qquad \text{(Eq. 6.7)}$$

Like Hammett values, Hansch's lipophilicity parameter, π, is based on how a substituent affects the position of an equilibrium. Hansch values specifically tell the effect of a substituent on the partitioning of a molecule between two solvents, typically water and 1-octanol (Fig. 6.2), as these two solvents have been found to closely model the membrane-aqueous interface in biological systems. The partitioning of the molecule between the two phases can be measured as equilibrium constant, *P* (Eq. 6.8). Using the octanol/water system, a whole series of partition coefficients were measured, and thus a new hydrophobic scale was introduced. The difference between the substituted and unsubstituted log *P* values gives the π value for that particular substituent (Eq. 6.9) thus, the π value for hydrogen is 0. As described for Hammett values, π values measure the free energy change caused by a particular substituent.

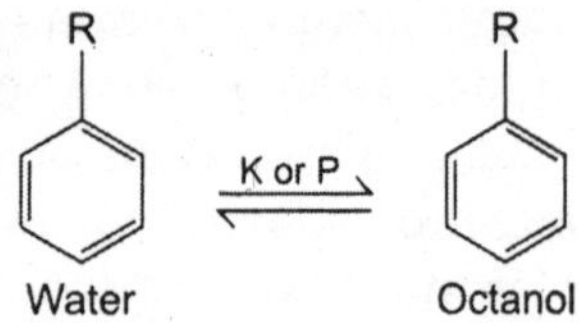

Fig. 6.2: Partitioning of a molecule between water and 1-octanol

$$P = \frac{(D_{\text{oct}})}{(D_{\text{water}})} \qquad \text{(Eq. 6.8)}$$

$$\pi_R = \log P_R - \log P_H \qquad \text{(Eq. 6.9)}$$

These σ and π values are measures of free energy changes, to relate them to the biological activity, biological activity must be somehow quantified in a form which is also related to free energy changes. Biological activity is often reported in terms of ED_{50} (dose/concentration required to achieve 50% of maximal response), IC_{50} (concentration required to achieve 50% inhibition), or LD_{50} (dose/concentration resulting in death of 50% of a population). As per the receptor theory, the values ED_{50}, IC_{50} and LD_{50} can be shown to be equal to the dissociation equilibrium constant of the drug and its receptor, K_D (Eq. 6.10). The logarithm of K_D is proportional to the free energy change of drug binding, so will be the logarithm of its equivalent such as IC_{50}, LD_{50}, etc. (Eq. 6.11). Values such as log IC_{50} are, therefore, useful in Hansch equations (Eq. 6.11) to try to relate to free energy parameters such as σ and π.

$$K_D = \frac{(\text{Receptor})(\text{Drug})}{(\text{Receptor-Drug})} \qquad \text{(Eq. 6.10)}$$

$$\log IC_{50} = \log K_D \; \alpha \Delta \text{G drug binding} \qquad \text{(Eq. 6.11)}$$

Hansch and Muir have published their brilliant study on the structure-activity relationships of plant growth regulators and their dependency on Hammett constants and hydrophobicity.

Fujita and Hansch then combined these hydrophobic constants with Hammett's electronic constants to yield the linear Hansch equation and its many extended forms, like Eq. 6.12.

$$\log 1/C = a\sigma + b\pi + ck \qquad \text{(Eq. 6.12)}$$

where C is molar concentration of the compound to produce a defined biological response, π is the hydrophobic contribution of the substituent, σ is Hammett electronic descriptor of the substituents.

Hundreds of equations later, the failure was observed with linear equations in cases with extended hydrophobicity ranges, this led to the development of the Hansch parabolic equation.

$$\log 1/C = a \log P - b (\log P)^2 + c\sigma + k \qquad \text{(Eq. 6.13)}$$

where, a and b are the coefficients of the log P and $(\log P)^2$.

The understanding of these models led to explosive development in QSAR analysis and related approaches. The Kubinyi's bilinear model is a refinement of the parabolic model and, in many cases, it has proved to be superior. Kubinyi made an important contribution in QSAR methodology in 1977 when he first proposed the bilinear model. In a large number of cases, it has been found that the biological activity increases with hydrophobicity linearly up to a certain point and then decreases in a linear fashion. The differences between observed and calculated biological activities were found to be high if parabolic models were used. The bilinear model to describe this nonlinear dependence of biological activity of drugs on hydrophobicity was expressed as:

$$\log 1/C = a \log P - b \log (\beta P + 1) + c \qquad \text{(Eq. 6.14)}$$

The terms a, b and c are linear in nature and can be calculated by multiple regression analysis whereas β is a nonlinear term and must be calculated by an iterative method. The introduction of Hansch's simple linear and parabolic models and Kubinyi's bilinear model made a considerable impact on our understanding of how chemical structures influence biological activity.

Free Wilson or *de novo* Method

Besides the Hansch approach, other scientists were trying to develop different methodologies to tackle structure-activity questions. The Free-Wilson approach is one such important approach; it is a general mathematical method for assessing the occurrence of additive substituent effects and for quantitatively estimating their magnitude. In this method the substituents are optimized within a molecular framework using the assumption that the introduction of a particular substituent at any one position in a molecule always changes the relative potency by the same amount, regardless of what other substituents are present in the molecule. It addresses structure-activity studies in a congeneric series as described in Eq. 6.15.

$$BA = ai\, xi + \mu \qquad \text{(Eq. 6.15)}$$

where *BA* is the biological activity, μ is the average contribution of the parent molecule, *ai* is the contribution of each structural feature; *xi* is given a value of one when the particular substituent is present or zero when it is absent.

Limitations in this approach led to the more sophisticated Fujita-Ban equation that used the logarithm of activity, which brought the activity parameter in line with other free energy-related terms.

$$\log BA = Ai\, Xi + \mu \qquad \text{(Eq. 6.16)}$$

where μ is defined as the calculated biological activity value of the unsubstituted parent compound of a particular series. *Ai* represents the biological activity contribution of the substituents, *Xi* denotes the presence ($Xi = 1$) or absence ($Xi = 0$) of a particular structural fragment. Variations on this activity-based approach have been extended by Klopman and Enslein.

Topological methods have also been used to address the relationships between molecular structure and physical/biological activity. The minimum topological difference (MTD) method of Simon and the extensive studies on molecular connectivity by Kier and Hall have contributed to the development of quantitative structure property/activity relationships. Connectivity indices based on hydrogen-suppressed molecular structures are rich in information on branching, 3-atom fragments, the degree of substitution, proximity of substituents and length, and heteroatom of substituted rings. A method in its embryonic state of development uses both graph bond distances and Euclidean distances among atoms to calculate *E*-state values for each atom in a molecule that is sensitive to conformational structure. Recently, these electrotopological indices that encode significant structured information on the topological state of atoms and fragments as well as their valence electron content have been applied to biological and toxicity data.

Apart from above discussed parameters/descriptors the development in this field has led to various ways of molecular representations which can be exemplified by molecular connectivity, topological and electrotopological indices, steric, lipophilic, electronic, quantum mechanical descriptors, molecular shapes, molecular fields, atomic counts, 2-*D* fragments, 3-*D* fragments, molecular eigen values, molecular multipole moments, *E*-state fields, molecular fragment-based hash codes and molecular holograms.

SOME MULTIVARIATE METHODS (OTHER APPROACHES)

In some cases biological activity values cannot be determined accurately using the above-mentioned procedures, for a variety of reasons, e.g. lack of sensitivity of a particular test system, huge data set, large number of descriptors, etc. Alternative statistical techniques can be used in these cases. Some of these techniques are defined below:

Cluster Analysis and Pattern Recognition Techniques

Pattern recognition methods attempt to define the set of parameter values which will result in clustering compounds of similar activity into regions of *n*-dimensional space.

The methods used to accomplish this goal can be parametric or nonparametric. Parametric methods search the n-dimensional space for clusters of compounds based on their calculated properties. These methods do not use derived values, e.g. mean vectors and covariance matrices, but instead use the original data to find clustering definitions and apply iterative procedures to find the linear set of parameters which best define the classification scheme. The compounds in a given set are labeled as active, partially active, inactive, etc. The resulting data set is then searched for patterns which predict these categories.

Jurs' group developed an alternate approach to examining the effects of chemical structure on activity. Rather than relying on multivariate statistics to highlight these relationships, they used the combination of cluster analysis and pattern recognition techniques as a tool to develop these correlations. They developed a program called ADAPT (Automated Data Analysis by Pattern recognition Techniques) which generated a data set of molecular descriptors (topological, geometrical and physicochemical) derived from three-dimensional model building, data points are then projected onto an n-dimensional surface and analyzed them using pattern recognition methods. The goal of this analysis was to discriminate between active and inactive compounds in a series. In one such study carried out by them on chemical carcinogens, 209 compounds from twelve structural classes (130 carcinogens, 79 non-carcinogens) were selected. Their structure features including fragment descriptors, substructure descriptors, environment descriptors, molecular connectivity descriptors and geometric descriptors were calculated. The program was used to identify a training set of 192 compounds which was used to find the best set of descriptors and analyze the entire data set. A predictive success of 90% for carcinogenic compounds and 78% for non-carcinogenic compounds was obtained in randomized testing.

The CASE (Computer-Automated Structure Evaluation) program extended the techniques in ADAPT by using topological methods to define sub-structural fragments which were essential for activity. CASE is able to differentiate between positional isomers. Both CASE and ADAPT are limited to analyzing structurally similar data sets. Another method which has been used for this type of analysis is CSA (Cluster Significance Analysis).

Principal Component Analysis (PCA)

PCA is a method, which is employed when the number of descriptors calculated for each structure in a data set is substantially more than the number of structures. It is probably the oldest and best-known technique of multivariate analysis. The central idea of the PCA is to reduce the dimensionality of a data set in which there are a large number of interrelated variables, while retaining as much as possible of the variation present in the data set. Thus, the objective of PCA is to create a reduced number variables which describe biological activity or chemical properties into a relatively few independent ones. This is accomplished through an analysis of the correlation matrix of biological or chemical properties. In this the descriptors are combined into smaller number of terms, called principal component, each of which is orthogonal to (i.e. uncorrelated with) the other. A typical PCA graph looks like Fig. 6.3.

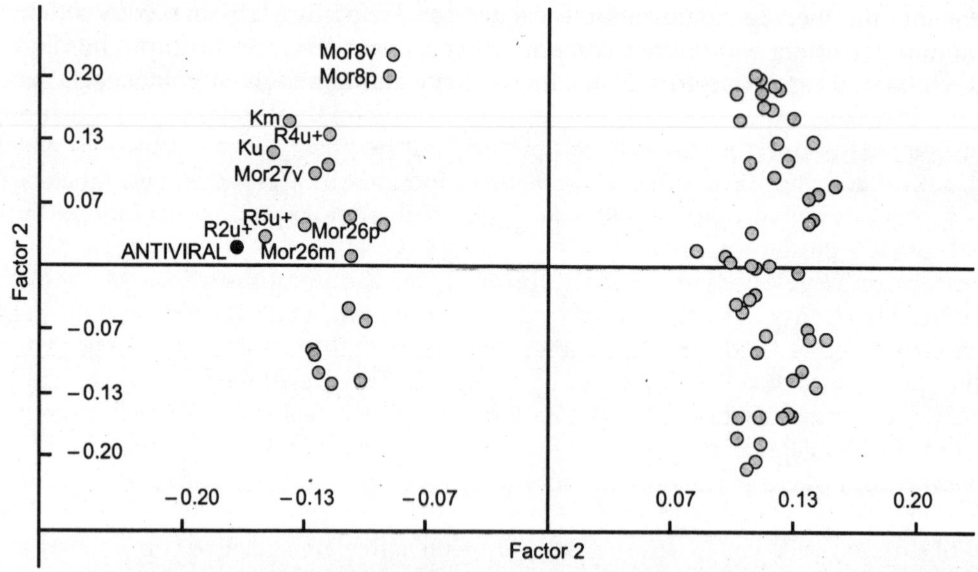

Fig. 6.3: PCA graph of a series of compounds with antiviral activity: The ● dot is showing the region in which antiviral activity is falling, and ○ dots are showing the descriptors. The principal components are those descriptors which are in the same region as activity.

The graph is divided into four zones, the descriptors which are lying in the region with the activity are the ones which are the principal components (i.e. highly correlated to the activity) and rest are orthogonal descriptors (i.e. uncorrelated with activity).

Principle component analysis can be used to create derived variables for each class (e.g. active and inactive) separately by decomposing the correlation matrix; this method is useful to point out redundancies or interrelationships among the variables. Using PCA we try to find simplified relationships in data by transforming the original parameters into a new set of uncorrelated variables which are termed principal components. The symmetric correlation matrix is decomposed by eigenvalue decomposition. The largest eigenvalue and its eigenvector are used to form a linear combination of the original variables with maximum variance. Successively smaller eigenvalues and vectors produce linear combinations of the original variables with lowering variance. Successive eigenvectors are independent of one another. The simplification of this can be done by omitting eigenvectors associated with small eigenvalues. In summary, the procedure finds the set of orthogonal axes for the data which decompose variance in the data.

SIMCA (Soft, Independent Modeling of Class Analogy) method uses Principal Component Analysis (PCA) to describe the data set.

Partial Least Square Analysis

Partial Least Square (PLS) analysis is a refinement of PCA. In this technique the principal component and the multiple regression analysis is done in a single step, and in addition to that, it is designed to give maximal correlation between the principal components and the dependent variable, e.g. biological activity. PLS can accommodate a large number of descriptors per compound, and is not adversely affected by high co-linearities among descriptors. Thus, it can easily accommodate large data sets.

Canonical Correlation Analysis

Canonical correlation analysis is a statistical technique that can be used to correlate simultaneously two or more different biological effects of the same set of the compounds.

3-D QSAR

In 1979, Marshall extended the 2-*D* approach to 3-*D* in QSAR by only considering the conformational flexibility of a series of structures as reflected by their 3-*D* shape, i.e. finding the active analogs. The first step of the *Active Analog Approach* is the exhaustive search of the conformations of a compound which is highly active in a particular biological assay. From this search we can obtain a map of interatomic distances of these active conformations, which can be used as a filter for conformational searches of subsequent molecules in the series. The major limitation of this method is the assumption that all compounds which display similar activity profiles are able to adopt similar conformations. Once the 'active conformation' was determined, molecular volumes for each molecule are calculated and superimposed. Regression analysis of these volumes is used to establish a relationship to biological activity. Marshall and co-workers commercialized the active analog approach and a suite of other drug design techniques in the SYBYL molecular modeling program.

Another group of scientists, Hopfinger and co-workers also used 3-*D* shape in QSAR around the same time. They performed *molecular shape analysis* of the Triazines, the common space shared by all molecules of a series and the differences in their potential energy fields were computed and combined with a set of rules for overlapping the series, comparative indicies of the shape of different molecules were obtained. These shape descriptors were included in standard Hansch analysis schemes, which led to improved descriptions relating computed parameters to biological activity. The techniques developed by Hopfinger were made available in the CAMSEQ, CAMSEQ-II, CHEMLAB and CAMSEQ-M computer programs.

In 1988, Richard Cramer proposed that biological activity could be analyzed by relating the shape-dependent steric and electrostatic fields for molecules to their biological activity. Thus, rather than limiting the analysis to fitting data to a regression line, *CoMFA (Comparative Molecular Field Analysis)* utilized new methods of data analysis, PLS (Partial Least Squares) and cross-validation, to develop models for activity predictions.

The approach used in the CoMFA procedure requires that the scientists define alignment rules for the series which overlap the putative pharmacophore for each molecule; the active conformation and alignment rule must be specified. Once aligned, each molecule is fixed into a three-dimensional grid by the program and the electrostatic and steric components of the molecular mechanics force field, arising from interaction with a probe atom (e.g. an sp^3 C atom) are calculated at intersecting lattice points within the 3-*D* grid. The equations which result from this exercise have the form

$$\text{Activity}_1 = \text{Constant}_1 + a_1\,(\text{steric}_{xyz}) + b_1\,(\text{steric}_{xyz}) + \ldots + a_1'\,(\text{estatic}_{xyz}) + b_1'\,(\text{estatic}_{xyz}) + \ldots$$

$$\text{Activity}_2 = \text{Constant}_2 + a_2\,(\text{steric}_{xyz}) + b_2\,(\text{steric}_{xyz}) + \ldots + a_2'\,(\text{estatic}_{xyz}) + b_2'\,(\text{estatic}_{xyz}) + \ldots$$

$$\text{Activity}_n = \text{Constant}_n + a_n\,(\text{steric}_{xyz}) + b_n\,(\text{steric}_{xyz}) + \ldots + a_n'\,(\text{estatic}_{xyz}) + b_n'\,(\text{estatic}_{xyz}) + \ldots$$

Traditional regression methods require that the number of parameters must be considerably smaller than the number of compounds in the data set (or the number of degrees of freedom in the data). The data tables which result from CoMFA analysis have far more parameters than compounds. PLS, which removes this limitation, is used to derive the coefficients for all of the steric and electrostatic terms. PLS essentially relies upon the fact that the correlations among near parts of a molecule are similar so that the real dimensionality is smaller than the number of grid points. Since these coefficients are position-dependent, substitution patterns for the series are elucidated which define regions of steric bulk and electrostatic charge associated with increase or decrease in the activity. The size of the model (the number of components needed for the best model) and the validity of the model as a predictive tool are assessed using cross-validation. Once a model is developed which has the highest cross-validated r^2, this model is used to derive the conventional QSAR equation and conventional r^2 and s values. The results of the final model are then visualized as contour maps of the coefficients. The first CoMFA study reported, analyzed the binding affinities of 21 steroid structures to human corticosteroid-binding globulins and testosterone-binding globulins.

Therefore, CoMFA starts with defined pharmacophore and overlap rules and derives a 3-*D* model which can be used to predict activity for new chemical entities. Whereas, the Apex and Catalyst (Accelrys, Formerly Molecular Simulations Incorporated) programs are used to identify pharmacophores from databases of chemical structures and biological activity. These models are then used to predict activities for novel compounds.

Apex-3-D is an automated pharmacophore identification system which can identify possible pharmacophores from a set of biologically active molecules using statistical techniques and 3-*D* pattern matching algorithms. The program classifies molecular structures using three steps:

- ***The agreement inductive method:*** It identifies common structural patterns in the given data set with similar activity;
- ***The difference inductive method:*** It identifies structural patterns which differentiate active and inactive compounds, and
- ***The concomitant variations inductive method:*** It highlights variations in structural features that explain changes in biological activity for sets of compounds.

To use this approach, the scientist is required to assign the training set of compounds to one or more activity classes; specific descriptor centers can also be defined if desired. The automated pharmacophore identification portion of the program then builds the knowledge base which can be used to predict biological activity for compounds not included in the training set.

The pharmacophores identified above can be used to build 3-*D* QSAR models by correlating indexes calculated for biophore sites, secondary sites or whole molecule properties. 3-*D* QSAR models in Apex are generated and screened using a modified scheme of multiple linear regression analysis with variable selection. Special randomization checks are made to estimate the chance of fortuitous correlation. The steps involved are:

- Interactively select the pharmacophore(s) to use in the analysis;
- Interactively choose parameters to include in the pool of possible parameters to be selected by the program, and
- Calculate the best 3-*D* QSAR models for each pharmacophore using stepwise multiple regression and analysis of statistics to assess the validity and predictive power of the model.

Using these 3-*D* QSAR models activities of novel compounds can be calculated based on each conformation which contains one of the pharmacophores and their fits in the model.

Catalyst is another software which generates structure-activity hypotheses from a set of molecules of various activities. Once molecular connectivity and activity values are specified for all molecules, Catalyst derives a hypothesis which consists of a set of generalized chemical functions (regions of hydrophobic surface, hydrogen bond vectors, charge centers, or other user-defined features) at specified relative positions. Up to ten hypotheses are produced and ranked by estimated statistical significance. The hypotheses can be examined graphically, fit to new molecules, or fed directly to flexible 3-*D* database search. The steps involved are:

- A set of representative conformers is found, that covers the low-energy conformational space of each molecule. Representative structures are chosen to maximize the sampling of conformational space.
- Locate a list of candidate hypotheses that are common among active and rare among inactive compounds (the presence of all identified features is not required for inclusion in the active class since it is unlikely that all active members of a training set possess all the important binding features).
- Statistical significance of the results (low probability of having found a chance correlation) on a variety of medicinal training sets is verified by a non-parametric randomization test.

Peter Goodford has reported an energy based GRID approach to compound design. The GRID program is a computational procedure for detecting energetically favorable binding sites on molecules of known structure. It has been used to study arrays of molecules in membranes and crystals or proteins. The energies are calculated as the electrostatic, hydrogen bond and Lennard-Jones interactions of a specific probe group with the target structure. GRID has also been used to distinguish between selective binding sites for different probes. In general, topological approaches start with a very different graph theoretic representation of molecular structure in which atoms are represented by vertexes and bonds by edges. Numerical indexes for the structure are then defined which abstract information including atom descriptors (atom types, atomic weight, atomic number, ratio of valance electrons to core electrons, etc.) and sub-group descriptors. In addition, a series of indexes (the χ indexes) are developed which describe the molecule as a set of fragments of varying size and complexity. Regression analysis of equations which have chi indexes as parameters has been used to correlate chemical structure to physicochemical behavior in applications such as chromatographic retention times, molar refractivity, ionization potential and heats of atomization. While the application of topological indicies has been widely reported in QSAR, the utility of these methods generally has been limited to predicting structure-property relationships for polymers and hydrocarbons.

Apart from the above-stated common software there are many more in the market which can be used for pharmacophore generation and 3-*D* QSAR. All these methods try to find out what pharmacophoric patterns are present in the active molecule which is not present in the inactive ones. Pharmacophores are defined by different chemical centers (atom-centered functional groups) and the distances between these centers. These descriptor centers can include such things as aromatic ring centers, electron donor ability, hydrogen bonding sites, lipophilic regions and partial atomic charge. The information for each molecule is stored in a knowledge base in the form of rules which can be used to predict the activity of novel structures. Pharmacophore and its role in drug designing is discussed separately in the next chapter.

NONLINEAR APPROACH

The goal of the QSAR modeling is to establish a trend in the descriptor values, which correlates either in a linear or nonlinear fashion, with the trend in biological activity. The development of combinatorial chemistry and high throughput screening technologies is leading to fast collection of structural and biological data. For these data 3-*D* method becomes quite expensive and secondly the linear correlation may not always hold true. For these considerations several non-linear QSAR methods have been proposed in last few years.

Most of these methods are based on artificial neural network (ANN) or machine learning techniques. *Artificial neural networks* (ANNs) is a comparatively recently developed field for QSAR. It has the ability to model non-rectilinear correlations, and thus can often model a data set better than MLR. To give valid results, it is essential for ANNs that they must be trained properly by using an appropriate training set. The main limitations are that they do not give regression equations and in the result the descriptors which have contributed to correlation are not indicated. An example is *k-Nearest Neighbor* (kNN) principle to QSAR (kNN-QSAR). The kNN-QSAR method employs multiple topological (2-*D*) or topographical (3-*D*) descriptors of chemical structures and predicts biological activity of any compound as the average activity of '*k*' most similar molecules. This method can be used for large data set.

The *Genetic Function Approximation* (GFA) algorithm is a novel technique for constructing QSAR models. It was specifically developed for use with data sets containing many more variables than samples, or data sets which contain nonlinear relationships between the variables and the activity. To begin with GFA in a population, we must have some randomly-constructed QSAR models; these models are checked for their predictive power, and then rated depending on the error in the measurement of relative predictiveness. The population is evolved by repeatedly selecting two better-rated models to serve as parents, then creating a new child model by using terms from each of the parent models. The worst-rated model in the population is replaced by this new model. As evolution proceeds, the population becomes enriched with higher and higher quality models.

The different models are, in effect, multiple fits to the data. Scientists can then use their scientific knowledge and intuition to select among the final models. Since the models usually use only a subset of the total number of variables in the data set, GFA behaves as a member of the class of variable reduction algorithms and is most useful if the critical information in the data set is concentrated in a few variables.

As evident from various research articles on the subject, GFA models were found to be comparable to, and in some cases superior to, models discovered using standard techniques such as stepwise regression, linear regression, or partial least-squares regression. With the increase in the number of computational and instrumentational sources of experimental data, the usefulness of GFA for performing variable reduction, discovering nonlinear relationships, and to present the user with multiple models representing multiple interpretations of the data set, will be more evident.

VALIDATION OF QSAR MODELS

The QSAR model developed by any of the above-mentioned methods does not hold any significance until it is validated, which means to check whether it has been proved to predict the property (activity) properly. To validate a QSAR model, i.e. to confirm its predictive performance; the available data set should be divided into the training set (TR) and test set (TS). Ideally the data set should be such divided that both the TR and TS should have full range of activity and they should be distributed such that the whole descriptor space is occupied by the both the sets.

To obtain the most reliable model in terms of predictive ability and robustness, the most popular tool is leave-one-out (LOO) or Leave-some-out (LSO). The results are shown in terms of cross validated r^2 (q^2), which is

$$q^2 = 1 - \frac{\Sigma\left(Y_i - \hat{Y}_i\right)^2}{\Sigma\left(Y_i - \bar{Y}_i\right)} \qquad \text{(Eq. 6.17)}$$

where, Y_i, $\hat{Y}_i$ and $\bar{Y}_i$ are the actual, estimated and averaged activities respectively.

A general method for the LOO method follows the following procedure:

- Eliminate one compound from the TR.

- Calculate the activity of the eliminated compound, as the average activity using the same set of descriptors.
- Repeat this procedure until every compound in the TR has been eliminated and predicted once.
- Calculate the cross-validated r^2 (q^2).
- Values for conventional r^2 range from 0 to 1. Values for the cross-validated r^2 are reported by the method to range from −1 to 1. Negative values indicate that biological activity values are estimated experimentally better than they are by the model, i.e. the predictions derived from the model are bad and should not be used.

Apart from binding there are many additional properties which contribute to the biological activity of a molecule including transportation, distribution, metabolism and elimination. Since the techniques described above address binding and typically do not account for any of these other processes, they often fail. However, one should note that their utility is one of efficiency and probability. They are generally more successful and efficient than are the mere scientific hunch/intuitive methods. Because no single method works for all cases, many groups are examining alternative approaches to developing SAR equations including electronic-based descriptors and topological indicies.

SUMMARY

Developing a quantitative structure activity relationship is difficult. Molecules are typically flexible and it is possible to compute many possibly useful properties that might relate to activity. Early in a research program there are typically few compounds to model. Thus, we have a few compounds in a very high dimensional descriptor space. Which are the important variables and how do we optimize them? It is clear that many training compounds need to span through the space and model fitting techniques need to address not only deriving a fit, but the predictive quality of the fit. While these methods have not discovered a new compound, they have aided scientists in examining the volumes of data generated in a research program. As the methods evolve, they will find broader application in areas such as combinatorial chemistry.

BIBLIOGRAPHY

1. Agarwal A, Pearson PP, Taylor EW, Li HB, Dahlgern T, Herslof M, Yang Y, Lambert G, Nelson DL, Regan JW and Martin AR, *J. Med. Chem.*, 1993, 36, 4006–4014.
2. Franke, R., In Theoretical Drug Design Methods, Elsevier, Amsterdam, 1984.
3. Hansch, C and Leo, A. in Heller, SR Ed., *Exploring QSAR. Fundamentals and Applications in Chemistry and Biology*, American Chemical Society, Washington, DC, 1995.
4. In *Burger's Medicinal Chemistry and Drug Discovery*, Burger A, Abraham, DJ, Andrako J, Block JH, Borchardt RT, Abraham Ed, 6th ed., Vol 5, A John Wiley and Sons, Inc., Publication: New Jersey, 2003.
5. John G. Topliss, Quantitative Structure–Activity Relationships of Drugs, Academic Press, New York, 1983.
6. Kubinyi H. Biological Activity on Hydrophobic Character: The Bilinear Model, II. Farmaco Ed (Sci), 1979; 34: 248–76.
7. Kier LB and Hall LH, *Molecular Connectivity in Chemistry and Drug Research*, Academic Press, New York, 1976 (28).

7 Pharmacophore-Based Drug Designing

INTRODUCTION

The rational development of pharmaceutical drugs is one major purpose of structural computational biology. Its goal is to make use of computational methods to aid in the design, discovery and optimization of new lead structures. The expectation is that computers will help in reducing the time, costs and resources that are required to get a new drug to the market. The two important aspects involved in predicting molecular interactions in computer-aided drug design (CADD) are pharmacophore-based and docking techniques. In the absence of a three-dimensional (3-*D*) structure of the receptor, only pharmacophore-based techniques are applicable. However, when this structure is available both pharmacophore-based and docking techniques can be applied. In particular, they can be employed synergistically integrated to improve the drug design process. Here, we review these two related aspects in the present and subsequent chapter. In this chapter we investigate the pharmacophore.

The term *pharmacophore* was first defined by Paul Ehrlich in 1909 as 'a molecular framework that carries (*phoros*) the essential features responsible for a drug's (*pharmacon's*) biological activity' (Ehrlich. *Dtsch. Chem. Ges.* 1909, 42: p.17). In 1977, this definition was updated by Peter Gund to 'a set of structural features in a molecule that is recognized at a receptor site and is responsible for that molecule's biological activity' (Gund. *Prog. Mol. Subcell. Biol.* 1977, 5: pp 117–143).

A pharmacophore is a specific, three-dimensional map of biological properties common to all active conformations of a set of ligands, which exhibit a particular activity, or it can be referred to as 3-*D* arrangement of the features that enable a molecule to exhibit a specific biological activity. In other words, molecules are active in a particular receptor if they carry a number of features that interact favorably with the receptor and which possess geometry complementary to it. Typical pharmacophore features for a molecule include hydrophobicity, aromaticity, a hydrogen bond acceptor, a hydrogen bond donor, a cation, or anion. These features are used to match different chemical groups with similar properties, in order to identify novel ligands. Ligand receptor interactions are typically 'polar positive', 'polar negative' or 'hydrophobic'. A well-defined pharmacophore model includes both hydrophobic volumes and hydrogen bond vectors.

Pharmacophores are conceptual templates for drug design. After the pharmacophore is identified it can be used to search a database of diverse set of more molecules which share the same features located at similar distance apart from each other. Once identified using a set of ligands possessing similar activity, a pharmacophore can be used as a model for the design of other molecules that can accomplish the same activity. The fact that most drug targets/receptors do not have established 3-*D* structures makes pharmacophore a more critical approach in virtual screening to identify novel inhibitors.

The importance of a pharmacophore in drug design is depicted in Fig. 7.1. It illustrates that there are two different ways to deduce a pharmacophore: *direct* methods and *indirect* methods. *Direct methods* use both ligand and receptor 3-D structure information. This approach plans an important rule in rational drug design. It is extensively used not only in drug lead optimization, but also in lead identification as long as several known inhibitors are available. Numerous software packages have been developed to generate pharmacophore models and to perform pharmacophore database searching today. Among these packages Phase, Galahad, Tuplets and Catalyst, are developed by utilizing three different algorithms which represent the latest development in the field.

The *indirect methods* use only a collection of ligands that have been experimentally observed to interact with a given receptor. Most of the times, the exact structure of the receptor is unknown. In such a situation, only indirect methods are applicable. However out of the two methods, the direct methods are becoming extremely important with the rapidly increasing number of known protein structures, which is the outcome of the structural genomics project. The various software available for the indirect approach are: DISCO, HIP-HOP, GASP, ChemX, GAMMA, RAPID, CLEW, etc.

Apart from using software, pharmacophore designing can be done using *Active Analog Approach* (AAA) and ensemble distance geometry. The analog-based pharmacophore can be generated either manually by visual pattern recognition or using AAA.

The AAA involves a systematic search of all the active ligands and then their rigid geometry approximation is done. The different fragments are screened and short-listed which bind to the receptor or contribute significantly towards the activity. The rigid body rotation is done and molecules are built

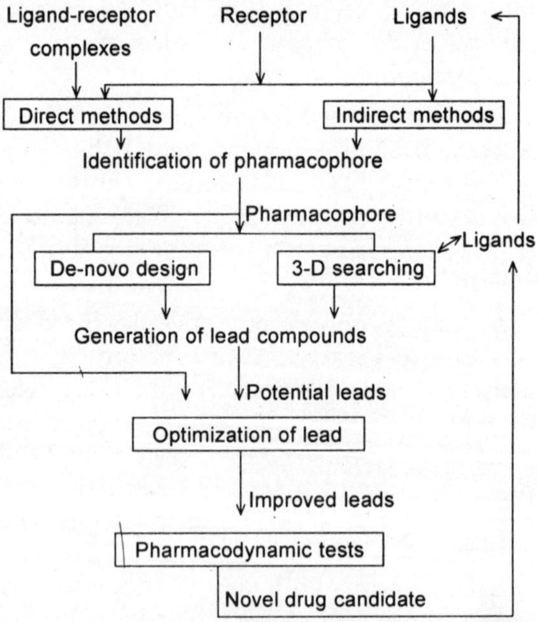

Fig. 7.1: Role of pharmacophore in drug designing

by aggregation. Some of the well-known examples of the application of *AAA* are Morphiceptin analoges, *ACE* inhibitors, Substance *P* antagonist.

Once identified, a pharmacophore model can be a versatile tool to aid in the discovery and development of new lead compounds. The power of pharmacophore-based methods for lead generation lies in their ability to suggest a diverse set of compounds potentially possessing a desired biological activity, but which have totally different chemical scaffolds. This is the main advantage of pharmacophore-based method over lead explosion, which usually generates a set of molecules that are very similar to the original lead and if a drug candidate fails because of ADME/toxicity reasons, similar candidates may also fail. Therefore, a diverse set of leads increases the chances that some of the compounds will pass all the stages of the drug development process. Alternatively, it can be used in *de novo* design, that is to develop totally new molecules that satisfy the pharmacophore requirements. Furthermore, a pharmacophore model can guide chemists to synthesize new compounds during lead optimization. Potential drug leads identified by such *in-silico* methods must be further verified by experimental tests. The results of the experimental tests provide useful information for the improvement of the pharmacophore model.

Applications of Pharmacophore

In this section we will see the applications of the generated pharmacophore that emphasize their usefulness.

- *Search of a New Pharmacophore*

Once identified, a pharmacophore model can often be used to identify novel pharmacologically active lead compounds by searching it against a database of known 3-D chemical structures like the ACD and CSD databases. This technique is known as lead identification or pharmacophore searching. Examples of such an application are well documented in literature. Pharmacophore searching methods use an identified pharmacophore as a query to screen 3-*D* databases of compounds. The result of this search is a set of compounds, called hits, which match the pharmacophore query. Some of these hits are similar to known active compounds, but some others may be entirely novel classes of compounds. Thus, pharmacophore searching can be useful in discovering novel lead compounds with different pharmacological properties. This diversity increases the chances that some of the compounds will pass all the stages of the drug development process.

Pharmacophore searching is part of a more general problem of 3-*D* structure searching, in which molecules in a database are examined to satisfy certain 3-*D* properties. In particular, these properties can be defined by the pharmacophore model. Therefore, many of the 3-*D* searching methods can be customized for the pharmacophore searching problem.

- *De Novo Design of Ligands*

The *de novo* design is the construction of novel ligands that satisfy the physicochemical parameters laid down by a given pharmacophore model. For example, in the

NEWLEAD method the input is given as a set of disconnected molecule fragments that are consistent with a pharmacophore model. Such input can be built from active ligands that are known to satisfy the pharmacophore. Then, these disjoint pharmacophoric fragments are linked to one another with connecting fragments that consist of small chemical groups (atoms, chains or ring moieties). If the structure of the receptor is known, one can use software packages like LUDI and BUILDER, which combine identification of receptor-based pharmacophore with *de novo* design.

De novo design and pharmacophore searching are two ways for lead generation. The difference between them is that by *de novo* design we can generate totally novel molecules, whereas pharmacophore searching identifies existing molecules, which can be easily obtained from databases of compounds. Thus, pharmacophore searching is faster and easier. However, in the absence of existing active ligands, only *de novo* design is applicable.

- *Lead Optimization*

Lead optimization is the process in which a biologically active compound is modified to fulfill all the properties that are required from a drug, e.g. physicochemical and ADME/Tox properties. It has been shown that a pharmacophore can direct us to include chemical functional features in the compounds synthesized during lead optimization. Lead optimization is a subsequent tool to lead generation. Specifically, the compounds synthesized during lead optimization are generally similar to the original leads, but they may have increased binding affinities to the desired target. In contrast, the compounds discovered or developed by a lead generation method (e.g. pharmacophore-based *de novo* design or pharmacophore searching) may be totally new compounds. These compounds display the pharmacophore and thus have a good chance of being bioactive, yet they may differ in other parts of the molecule.

- *In 3-D QSAR*

As discussed in the previous chapter, 3-*D* Quantitative Structure Activity Relationships (QSAR) analyses the correlation between the structural features and the biological activity in order to predict the activity level of new compounds. Using statistical correlation methods, it builds models to predict quantities such as binding affinity, toxicity, or pharmacokinetic parameters of existing or hypothetical molecules. 3-*D* QSAR analyses the three-dimensional forces like hydrogen bonds, metal-ligand contacts, polarization effect and the interaction between the electric dipoles. Obtaining a correct superimposition between the input ligand molecules is one of the first and most crucial stages of QSAR analysis, which has a strong impact on the reliability of the derived QSAR model. Pharmacophore models reflect an ideal geometry of the alignment of pharmacophoric elements (in the absence of steric hindrances and constraints due to internal energy) and, therefore, can be used to generate good alignments useful for QSAR analysis.

Summary

Pharmacophores play a key role in computer-aided drug design, especially in the absence of a receptor structure. The power of pharmacophore-based methods for drug design lies in their ability not only to suggest a diverse set of compounds having a potential to possess a desired biological activity, but those also which have totally different chemical scaffolds. However, the major limitation associated with a pharmacophore approach is that several pharmacophores may be possible within a single binding site and one pharmacophore may not describe all the possible ligands. In addition, at times receptor may have more than one active site. In such situations it becomes important to distinguish between them and construct two or more different pharmacophores. Furthermore, we must remember that a pharmacophore is a necessary but not the only condition for the ligand to interact at the receptor site; other factors like transport properties and size must also be considered.

BIBLIOGRAPHY

1. Davies K, Upton R. 3-*D* pharmacophore searching, Online available at *http://www.netsci.org/Science/Cheminform/feature02.html.*
2. Dror O, Shulman-Peleg A, Nussinov R, Wolfson HJ. *Curr Med Chem.* 2004, 11 (1): 71–90.
3. Guner OF, Henry DR. Three-dimensional Structure Searching. In Encyclopedia of Computational Chemistry, Schleyer PVR, Allinger NL, Clark T, Gasteiger J, Kollman PA, Schaefer III, HF, Schreiner PR, Eds John Wiley & Sons: Chichester, UK: , 1998.
4. Kubinyi H. Comparative Molecular Field Analysis (CoMFA). In Encyclopedia of Computational Chemistry; Schleyer PVR, Allinger NL, Clark T, Gasteiger J, Kollman PA, Schaefer III, HF, Schreiner PR, Eds.; John Wiley & Sons: Chichester, UK:, 1998.
5. Leclerc F, Cedergren R. Structure–Activity Relationships in Modeling Nucleic Acid Ligand Interactions. In Encyclopedia of Computational Chemistry; Schleyer PVR, Allinger NL; Clark T, Gasteiger J, Kollman PA, Schaefer III, HF, Schreiner PR, Eds; John Wiley & Sons: Chichester, UK:, 1998.
6. Marriott DP, Dougall IG, Meghani P, Liu YJ, Flower DRJ. *Med. Chem.* 1999, 42, 3210–3216.
7. Marshall G, Barry C, Bosshard H, Dammkoehler R, Dunn D. The Conformational Parameter in Drug Design: The Active Analog Approach. In Computer-Assisted Drug Design, Vol. 112; Olson E, Christoffersen R, Eds; ACS, Washington, DC, 1979.
8. Milne, GMA. Pharmacophore and Drug Discovery. In Encyclopedia of Computational Chemistry; Schleyer PR, Allinger NL, Clark T, Gasteiger J, Kollman PA, Schaefer III, HF, Schreiner PR, Eds; John Wiley & Sons: Chichester, UK:, 1998.
9. Paris CG. Structure Databases. In Encyclopedia of Computational Chemistry; Schleyer PVR, Allinger NL, Clark T, Gasteiger J, Kollman PA, Schaefer III, HF, Schreiner PR, Eds; John Wiley & Sons: Chichester, UK:, 1998.
10. Sheridan R, Nilakantan R, Dixon J, Venkataraghavan, RJ. *Med. Chem.* 1986, 29, 899–906.
11. Walters WP, Stahl MT, A MM. High throughput 'Virtual' Chemistry. In Encyclopedia of Computational Chemistry; Schleyer PVR, Allinger NL, Clark T, Gasteiger J, Kollman PA, Schaefer III, HF, Schreiner PR, Eds; John Wiley & Sons: Chichester, UK:, 1998.
12. Wang S, Zaharevitz D, Sharma R, Marquez V, Lewin N, DU L, Blumberg P, Milne GJ. *Med. Chem.* 1994, 37, 4479–4489.

8 Molecular Docking

INTRODUCTION

The rapid accumulation of three-dimensional structures of protein complexes through X-ray crystallization is amongst the many recent advances in bioinformatics. These structures provide many insights on protein-protein or ligand (drug)-protein interactions, allowing more rational approaches towards drug development and the treatment of disease. Most of the times data are available for the shape of a protein and a drug separately, but not for the two bound together. *Docking* is the process by which two molecules fit together in 3-*D* space. By this method we can predict the preferred orientation of one molecule to a second when bound to each other to form a stable complex. This knowledge of the preferred orientation in turn may be used to predict the strength of association or binding affinity between two molecules (i.e. drug and receptor) for example, by using scoring functions.

Molecular docking can be defined as an optimization problem, which would describe the 'best-fit' orientation of a ligand that binds to a particular protein of interest (Fig. 8.1). However, since both the ligand and the protein are flexible, a *hand-in-glove* analogy is more appro-priate than *lock-and-key* where the protein is analogous to the glove and the ligand is analogous to hand which will go and fit into the protein. During the process of binding, the ligand and the protein adjust their conformation to achieve an overall 'best-fit' and this kind of conformational adjustments resulting in the overall binding is referred to as 'induced-fit'. Docking is used to predict the binding orientation of small molecule drug candidates to their protein targets in order to predict the affinity

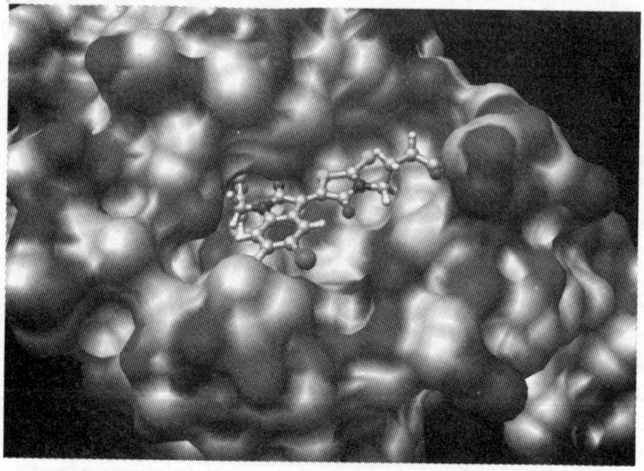

Fig. 8.1: A molecule begin docked into the active site of the protein

and activity of the small molecule. Hence, docking plays an important role in the rational design of drugs.

The associations between biologically relevant molecules such as proteins, nucleic acids, carbohydrates and lipids play a key role in signal transduction. Furthermore, the relative orientation of the two interacting partners may affect the type of signal produced, e.g. agonism vs. antagonism. Therefore, docking is useful for predicting both the strength of binding and type of signal produced.

Given the biological and pharmaceutical significance of molecular docking, considerable efforts have been directed towards improving the methods used to predict docking.

There are certain terms that are specific for molecular docking:

- ***Receptor:*** The receiving molecule that primarily binds to a small molecule or another protein or a nucleic acid.
- ***Ligand:*** A molecule that forms the complementary partner in the docking process. It is usually the molecule/drug designed to dock in the receptor.
- ***Pose:*** A conformation of the receptor and ligand molecules showing some intermolecular interactions (which may include hydrogen bonds as well as hydrophobic contacts).
- ***Posing:*** The process of searching for a pose in which there are favorable interactions between the receptor and the ligand molecules.
- ***Scoring:*** The process of evaluating a particular pose using a number of descriptive features like number of intermolecular interactions including hydrogen bonds and hydrophobic contacts.
- ***Ranking:*** The process of classifying which of the ligands bind favorably to a particular receptor, evaluating and analyzing free energy of binding.

The centre of attention of molecular docking is to computationally stimulate the process of molecular recognition, i.e. how a receptor and the ligand recognize and adapt themselves to accommodate each other. The aim of molecular docking is to achieve an optimized conformation for both the protein and ligand and relative orientation between protein and ligand such that the free energy of the overall system is minimized.

Approaches to Molecular Docking

There are two approaches that are particularly popular in the molecular docking. One approach uses a matching technique that describes the protein and the ligand as complementary surfaces. The second approach simulates the actual docking process in which the ligand-protein pairwise interaction energies are calculated. Both approaches have significant advantages as well as some limitations. These are outlined below.

- ***Geometric matching:*** In geometric matching/shape complementarity methods, the protein and ligand are described as a set of features that make them dockable. These features may include molecular surface/complementary surface descriptors. In this case, the receptor's molecular surface is described in terms of its surface area that is accessible to the solvent, and the ligand's molecular surface is described in terms of how much it matches that surface description. The complementarity between the two surfaces amounts to the shape matching description that may help finding the complementary pose of docking the target and the ligand molecules. Another approach is to describe the hydrophobic features of the protein using turns in the main-chain atoms. Yet another approach is to use a Fourier shape descriptor technique described by Shoichet BK, et. al. Whereas the shape complementarity-based approaches are typically fast and robust, they cannot take into account the movements or dynamic changes in the ligand/protein conformations accurately, although recent developments allow these methods to investigate ligand flexibility. Shape complementarity methods can quickly scan through several thousand ligands in a matter of seconds and actually figure out whether they can bind at the protein's active site, and are usually scalable to even protein-protein interactions. They are also much more agreeable to pharmacophore-based approaches, since they use geometric descriptions of the ligands to find optimal binding.

- ***Simulation process:*** The simulation of the docking process is a much more complicated process. In this approach, the protein and the ligand are separated by some physical distance, and the ligand finds its position into the protein's active site after a certain number of 'moves' in its conformational space. The moves incorporate rigid body transformations like translations and rotations, as well as internal changes to the ligand's structure including torsion angle rotations. Each of these moves made by the ligand to fit into the active site of receptor possesses a particular amount of energy, and hence, after every move the total energy of the system is calculated. The main advantage of the method is that it is more open to incorporate ligand flexibility into its modeling. Another advantage is that the process is physically closer to what happens in reality, when the protein and ligand approach each other after molecular recognition. The disadvantage of this technique is that it takes longer time to evaluate the optimal pose of binding since they have to explore a rather large energy landscape. However, grid-based techniques as well as fast optimization methods have significantly lowered these problems.

Some of the popular docking softwares are: Auto dock, FT (Fourier transform) Dock, RP (Residula level pair potential) Score and Multi (Multiple copy side-chain refinement) Dock, ZDOCK, RDOCK, Docking@GRID, Paradiseo@GRID, HADDOCK (High Ambiguity-driven biomolecular docking, based on biochemical and/or biophysical information), Quantum, Surflex-dock, Benchware Dock, etc.

The Mechanics of Docking

To perform a docking screen, the first requirement is a structure of the protein of interest, which is usually obtained by X-ray crystallography or protein data bank. This protein structure and a database of potential ligands serve as inputs to a docking program. The success of a docking program depends on two components: the search algorithm and the scoring function.

Search algorithm: Searching the conformational space for docking.

Search space is the space, which consists of all possible orientations and conformations of the protein paired with the ligand. Using the presently available computing resources, it is impossible to exhaustively explore the search space that includes listing all possible distortions of each molecule (molecules are dynamic and exist in an ensemble of conformational states) and all possible rotational and translational orientations of the ligand relative to the protein. Most docking programs in use account for ligand flexibility, and several are attempting to model a flexible protein receptor. Each 'snapshot' of the pair is referred to as a pose. There are many strategies for sampling the search space. Here are some examples:

- Use a coarse-grained molecular dynamics simulation to propose energetically reasonable poses.
- Use a 'linear combination' of multiple structures determined for the same protein to emulate receptor flexibility.
- Use a genetic algorithm to 'evolve' new poses that are successively more and more likely to represent favorable binding interactions.

Scoring Function

The scoring function takes a pose as input and returns a number which indicates the likelihood that the pose represents a favorable binding interaction. Most scoring functions are physics-based molecular mechanics force fields that estimate the energy of the pose; a low (negative) energy indicates a stable system and thus a likely binding interaction. An alternative approach is to derive a statistical potential for interactions from a large database of protein-ligand complexes, such as the Protein Data Bank, and evaluate the fit of the pose according to this inferred potential.

There are a lot of structures from X-ray diffraction for complexes between proteins and high affinity ligands, but for low affinity ligands these structures are very few because these do not stay bound for long enough to be seen. Scoring functions trained with this data can dock high affinity ligands correctly, but they will also give reasonable docked conformations for ligands that are really inactive. This gives a large number of false positive hits, i.e. ligands predicted to bind to the proteins that actually do not when placed together in a test tube.

One way to reduce the number of false positives is to recalculate the energy of the top-hit poses using a higher resolution (and therefore slow) technique like Generalized Born or Poisson-Boltzmann methods. However, typically the researcher will screen a database of tens to hundreds of thousands of compounds and test the top 60 or so *in vitro*, and to identify any true binders is still considered a success.

Applications

A binding interaction between a small molecule ligand and an enzyme protein may result in activation or inhibition of the enzyme. If the protein is a receptor, ligand binding may result in agonism or antagonism. Docking is most commonly used in the field of drug design—most drugs are small organic molecules, and docking may be applied to:

- ***Hit identification:*** Docking combined with a scoring function can be used to quickly screen large databases of potential drugs in silico to identify molecules that are likely to bind to protein target of interest (see virtual screening).
- ***Lead optimization:*** Docking can be used to predict where and in which relative orientation a ligand binds to a protein (also referred to as the binding mode or pose). This information may in turn be used to design more potent and selective analogs.

BIBLIOGRAPHY

1. Feig M, Onufriev A, Lee MS, Im W, Case DA, Brooks CL (2004). Performance comparison of generalized born and Poisson methods in the calculation of electrostatic solvation energies for protein structures. *Journal of Computational Chemistry* 25 (2): 265–84.
2. Jorgensen WL (1991). Rusting of the lock and key model for protein-ligand binding. *Science* 254 (5034): 954–5. Shoichet BK, Kuntz ID, Bodian DL (2004). Molecular docking using shape descriptors. *Journal of Computational Chemistry* 13 (3): 380–397.
3. Kitchen DB, Decornez H, Furr JR, Bajorath J (2004). Docking and scoring in virtual screening for drug discovery: methods and applications. *Nature reviews. Drug discovery* **3** (11): 935–49.
4. Lengauer T, Rarey M (1996). Computational methods for biomolecular docking. *Curr. Opin. Struct. Biol.* 6 (3): 402–6.
5. Meng EC, Shoichet BK, Kuntz ID (2004). Automated docking with grid-based energy evaluation. *Journal of Computational Chemistry* 13 (4): 505–524.
6. Morris GM, Goodsell DS, Halliday RS, Huey R, Hart WE, Belew RK, Olson AJ (1998). Automated docking using a Lamarckian genetic algorithm and an empirical binding free energy function. *Journal of Computational Chemistry* 19 (14): 1639–1662.
7. Wei BQ, Weaver LH, Ferrari AM, Matthews BW, Shoichet BK (2004). Testing a flexible-receptor docking algorithm in a model binding site. *J. Mol. Biol.* 337 (5): 1161–82.

9 UV Spectrophotometry

INTRODUCTION

The term photometry indicates measurement of light or its properties. In accordance with this meaning, a spectrophotometer is meant to be a device that measures the intensity of light. There are many kinds of spectrophotometers that can measure intensity as a function of color or more specifically, the wavelength of light. Spectrophotometers are classified according to the light sources used, the range of their working wavelengths, the measurement techniques used, the method of acquiring a spectrum, etc. In pharmacy, there are many applications of spectrophotometers. Perhaps the most common application of spectrophotometers is the measurement of light absorption, but they can be designed to measure the reflected light too.

A UV spectrometer usually measures the intensity of light. Most of the drugs are complex molecules having one or more groups endowed with the power of light absorption. Hence, spectrophotometric techniques are widely used in pharmacy for the purpose of identification as well as quantification of drug substances. Numbers of instruments have been designed on the basis of light absorption. The instruments vary according to the complexity and accuracy of measurement. They may range from the simplest 'Flame photometer' and 'Colorimeter' to the most sophisticated 'Atomic absorption spectrometer' and 'Mass spectrophotometer'. However, of all types of spectrophotometry, UV spectrophotometry is the most widely used in pharmacy as most drugs absorb radiation in the ultraviolet region of the spectrum. This chapter introduces the basics of UV spectrophotometry.

Advantages associated with a UV spectrophotometer:

- Simplicity of operation.
- Ease of maintenance.
- Cost effectiveness.
- High sensitivity (microgram and nanogram levels can be measured).
- Needs little or no pretreatment of samples.

Disadvantages: UV spectrophotometers usually measure the light as a whole, restricting its utility in the measurement of pure or binary mixture. The device cannot differentiate between the light lost or gained due to different causes. For this reason, assay of active ingredients from pharmaceutical dosage forms are often done by HPLC, where column separates the components of the sample mixture before quantification is done by UV absorption property.

Molecular spectra: Molecules are usually complex entities containing more than one atom. Drugs are complex molecules having different types of atoms bonded together with the potential of widespread absorption. Hence, molecules can undergo a large number of transitions. Molecular absorption in the ultraviolet and visible region is dependent on the electronic structure of the molecule. However, many electronic structures do not absorb in the UV region and UV absorption is normally limited to conjugated systems. The molecules absorb energy provided by light and undergo electronic (jumping of the electron to the higher energy orbital), vibrational and rotational transitions.

Beer-Lambert's Law

When light passes through a solution of light-absorbing species, some of the light is lost during the passage and some of it gets transmitted. Hence, the intensity of transmitted light is usually lesser than the incident light. In both UV and visual spectrophotometry, quantum of the light absorbed is measured and related to the concentration of absorbing species in solution.

The solution is kept in a transparent container called cell or cuvette. During passage, in addition to the solution, light has to pass through the walls of the cuvette and some light may be absorbed or reflected by the materials of the cuvette too. For accuracy of measurement, it is necessary to neutralize these parallel sources of absorption.

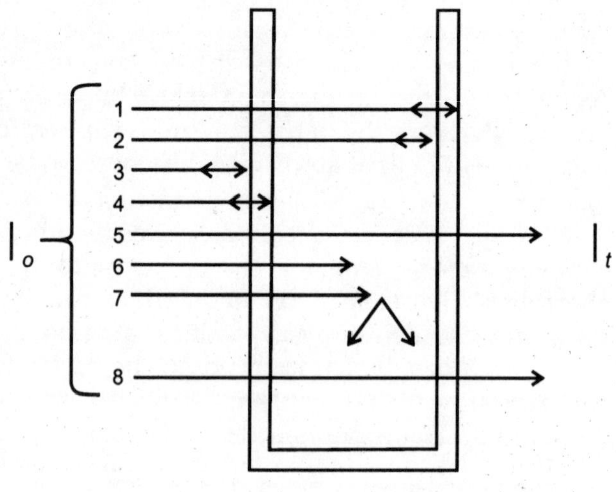

Fig. 9.1: Schematic representation of transmission of light through a drug solution

In Fig. 9.1, we have numerically marked the light rays, which are directed to the solution kept in a cuvette. It is seen that out of 8 rays, only 2 have passed through the solution and the intensity of transmitted light is much lesser than the incident light.

The reduction in the intensity of light has occurred due to

(*a*) Reflection by the inner and outer surfaces of the cuvette (rays 1–4).

(*b*) Scatter by particles in solution (ray 7).

(*c*) Absorption by molecules of the solution (ray 6).

Usually, the objective of UV spectrophotometry is to quantify the absorption caused by a desired analyte. This is done by subtracting the absorption of the solvent and other sources from the total absorbance.

The reflection at the cell surfaces is compensated by using a reference cell containing the solvent that ensures the loss of same amount of light and the scatter is neutralized by filtering the solution. The basic principle is

$$I_{\text{absorbed}} = I_0 - I_T \quad \text{(Eq. 9.1)}$$

Here, I_0 is the incident light and I_T, the transmitted light.

Beer-Lambert's law, which is the combination of two laws framed by two scientists describes the ratio of the incident light to the transmitted light as a function of pathlength and concentration of the absorbing species.

Lambert's Law

The Lambert's law was framed first. Back in 1760, Lambert had discovered that the intensity of a beam of parallel monochromatic light decreases exponentially as it passes through a medium of homogeneous thickness. Simply stated, absorbance was found to be proportional to the length of the path it passes through.

Mathematically, the relationship is described as

$$-\frac{dI}{db} \propto I$$

Here, dI represents the decrease in intensity of light while passing through a medium of thickness db.

$$\therefore \quad -\frac{dI}{db} = K'I$$

Here, I represents the intensity of light and K', the proportionality constant. Taking reciprocal of both sides, we get,

$$-\frac{db}{dI} = \frac{1}{K'I}$$

On integration the expression becomes,

$$-b = \frac{\ln I_T}{K'} + C \quad \text{(Eq. 9.2)}$$

where I_T is the transmitted radiation.

When $b = 0$, i.e. the thickness of the layer through which the light passed is assumed 0, I_T becomes I_0.

$$\therefore \quad C = -\frac{\ln I_0}{K'}$$

Substituting the value of C in Eq. 9.2.

$$-b = \frac{1}{K'}\ln I_T - \frac{1}{K'}\ln I_0$$

$$\therefore \qquad \ln \frac{I_T}{I_0} = -K'b$$

On changing sides the expression becomes,

$$\log \frac{I_0}{I_T} = \frac{K'b}{2.303}$$

Absorbance is defined as

$$\log \frac{I_0}{I_T}.$$

The terms extinction and optical density are also used for it.

As Lambert's law gives the relationship of absorbance with pathlength of absorption process, Beer's law gives the relationship of absorbance with the concentration of the absorbing species. The intensity of transmitted light decreases exponentially with the increase in concentration of absorbing species. The relationship is described as

$$\log \frac{I_0}{I_T} = \frac{K''C}{2.303}.$$

Where C represents concentration and K'' is the proportionality constant.

Beer-Lambert's law is a combination of these two laws and the combination rate constant of $K'/2.303$ and $K''/2.303$ is represented as absorptivity (a).

So the final expression is $\log \frac{I_0}{I_T} = abc.$

Where a is the absorptivity, b is the pathlength and c represents the concentration of the absorbing species.

The more popular form of this expression is

$$A = \varepsilon c l \qquad \text{(Eq. 9.3)}$$

Where,

A = absorbance,

ε = molar absorptivity,

c = concentration,

l = pathlength of light.

Some Important Terms and Concepts

Absorptivity: Absorptivity is a measure of intensity of absorption. The value of absorptivity depends on the units of concentration used for the absorbing solution. It can be expressed in percentage (E 1%, 1 cm) or molar absorptivity (ε).

Molar absorptivity: It is the absorbance of 1 M solution of a substance when the pathlength of light (width of cuvette) is 1 cm. Molar absorptivity is expressed with the symbol ε (epsilon). The use of molar absorptivity as a unit of absorption has one advantage. Absorbance of various species can be compared as all absorption values refer to the same number of absorbing species.

Specific absorbance: It is the absorbance of 1% solution with a pathlength of 1 cm. Specific absorbance is expressed as $A^{1\%}_{1cm}$. Specific absorbance can be converted into molar absorptivity by using the following relationship.

$$\varepsilon = \frac{A^{1\%}_{1cm} \times \text{mol. wt}}{10} \qquad \text{(Eq. 9.4)}$$

UV spectrum: A UV spectrum is simply a plot of wavelength of absorption versus the absorption intensity. Since UV energy is quantized, the absorption spectra due to a single electronic transition should have a single line. But such discrete lines are not obtained, as electronic absorption is superimposed on rotational and vibration sublevels. In molecules with many atoms, many vibrational sublevels exist in close proximity with each other and hence, instead of sharp lines, we get broad absorption bands. The relative energies of electronic: vibrational: rotational transitions are 100 : 1 : 0.01. In most molecules, the vibrational behaviour is complex and different energies of the vibrational transitions overlap partially, making the identification of fine structures difficult. The transition from single ground state energy to a number of excited states gives width to the UV spectra.

Bathochromic shift: The shift of absorption to higher wavelength due to solvent or substitution effect is called bathochromic or red shift. The red shift presumably results from a reduction in energy levels of the excited state along with dipole-dipole interaction and hydrogen bonding.

Hypsochromic shift: It is the opposite of bathochromic effect. Shift of absorption to shorter wavelength due to solvent or substitution is called hypsochromic shift.

Hyperchromic shift: An increase in the absorption intensity is known as hyperchromic shift.

Hypochromic shift: A decrease in absorption intensity is known as hypochromic shift.

Natural bandwidth and λ_{max}: If the absorbance of a species is measured at different wavelengths, it is seen that absorption at certain section of the spectrum increases gradually to reach the maximum value then falls again. The wavelength at which peak absorption is recorded is called λ_{max}. The width of the absorption band at one-half of the λ_{max} is defined as the natural bandwidth of the absorbing species (Fig. 9.2).

It is shown that if the spectral bandwidth is greater than 1/10th of its natural bandwidth, λ_{max} recorded will be lesser than its true value.

Chromophores: The term chromophore is usually used to mean extended system of double bonds, which are the groups responsible for electronic transition. The most common chromophore found in a drug molecule is benzene ring. Benzene shows a broad absorption band containing multiple peaks or fine structure in the near UV region (230 to 270 nm). When a chromophoric group is attached to an aromatic ring, absorption bands are observed at higher wavelengths.

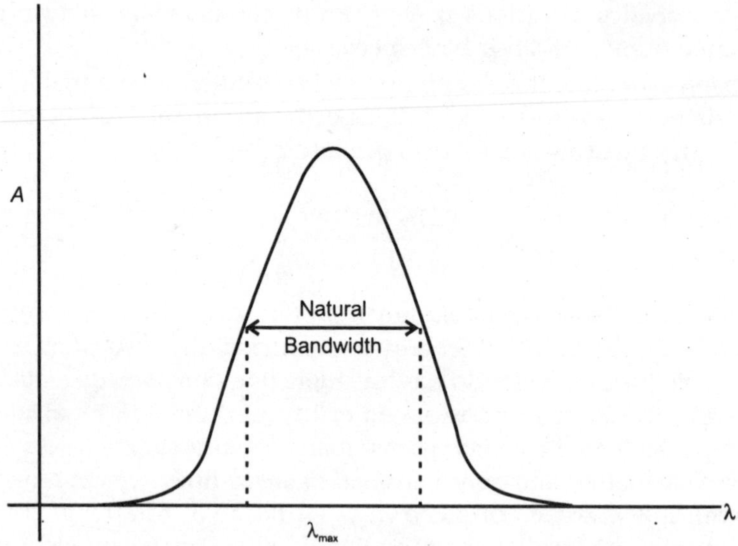

Fig. 9.2: The natural bandwidth of an ideal absorption band

Single chromophoric groups like C = O, NO_2 have low molar absorptivity (<100). With increased polarity of the solvent, they show a hypsochromic shift. Molecules having conjugated systems can undergo transitions. Such molecules typically have high molar absorptivity. Spectra of such molecules are also unaffected by the solvent polarity as hydrocarbon double bonds are nonpolar in nature.

Auxochrome: Auxochromes are saturated groups with nonbonded electrons. Auxochromes, attached to a chromophore, can modify the wavelength as well as intensity of absorption, e.g. OH, NH_2, Cl, etc.

Spectrophotometers: There are two major classes of spectrophotometers: single beam and double beam. A single beam spectrophotometer measures the absolute light intensity whereas the double beam spectrophotometer measures the ratio of the light intensity on two different light paths (Fig. 9.3).

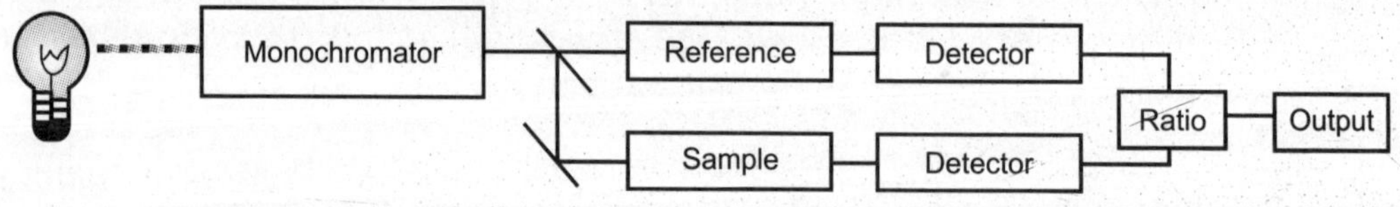

Fig. 9.3: Schematic diagram of a spectrophotometer

Various Parts of a Spectrophotometer

Light source: To generate the light that is to be absorbed by the solution, spectrophotometers must have a light source. The wavelengths of light obtained from a light source depend on its temperature; the higher the temperature, the shorter the wavelength of peak emission. However, a light source can be heated up to a certain point only. If overheated, metals can melt and volatilize causing a lamp burn out. It is also important that the power of the radiation source does not undergo abrupt change over its wavelength range.

Tungsten filament lamp: Tungsten filaments emit light in the range of 350 to 2000 nm. Like an ordinary light bulb, the tungsten filament is covered in a glass covering. The life of this lamp depends on the rate of evaporation of tungsten. As tungsten evaporates with time, the inside of the envelope becomes darker and energy of the incident light reduces.

Tungsten-halogen lamp: Tungsten-halogen lamps contain a small amount of iodine in quartz envelope, which also contains the tungsten filament. The iodine reacts with gaseous tungsten, formed by sublimation, producing the volatile compound WI_2. When molecules of WI_2 hit the filament they decompose, re-depositing tungsten back on the filament. The lifetime of a tungsten-halogen lamp is approximately double to that of an ordinary tungsten filament lamp. Tungsten-halogen lamps are very efficient, and their output extends well into the ultra violet region. Halogen (iodine) prevents evaporation of the tungsten and extends the life of the lamp.

Deuterium lamp: A deuterium discharge lamp consists of two electrodes in a deuterium filled silica envelope. High voltage is applied to these electrodes through a special power supply. As powerful current passes through the electrodes, deuterium lines are emitted. The lines are absorbed by deuterium (within the bulb) and a continuous spectrum of light within the range of 185 to 380 nm is emitted. The electrical excitation of deuterium or hydrogen at low pressure produces a continuous UV spectrum. The mechanism for this emission involves formation of an excited molecular species, which breaks up to give two atomic species and an ultraviolet photon. The reaction can be shown as,

$$D_2 + \text{electrical} - \text{energy} \rightarrow D_2^* \rightarrow D' + D'' + h\nu.$$

Both deuterium and hydrogen lamps emit radiation in the range 160–375 nm. Below 185 nm, the intensity of light is reduced by absorption of silica. Deuterium lamps have a lifespan 5 times higher than that of hydrogen lamps.

Wavelength selector (monochromator): Light produced by the light sources of a spectrophotometer is mixtures of many wavelengths. Since the absorbing moieties have different affinity for different wavelengths, for measurement of absorption intensity, lights of specific wavelengths are supplied. Monochromators are the devices, which disperse the incident light to create monochromatic light. All monochromators contain the following component parts. An entrance slit, a collimating lens, a dispersing device (usually a prism or a grating), a focusing lens and an exit slit.

Polychromatic radiation (radiation of more than one wavelength) enters a monochromator through the entrance slit. The beam is collimated, and then strikes the dispersing element at an angle where it is split into its component wavelengths by the grating or prism. By moving the dispersing element, radiation of only a particular wavelength can be selected to pass through the exit slit.

Filter: Filters absorb certain wavelengths while allowing others to pass through it. A filter absorbing yellow light appears blue. In photometry, filters are used to block certain lights and selectively transmit others.

Prisms: An optical prism is a transparent body, with usually three rectangular plane faces or sides used for dispersing light. Prisms, made of quartz are used to disperse light in ultraviolet spectrophotometers. Glass absorbs light of wavelengths lower than 330 nm and hence, glass prisms are used in visual spectrophotometer.

Grating: In the modern spectrophotometers, gratings are the devices used for dispersing light. The dispersing element in monochromator is diffraction grating. It is basically a glass plate or light transmitting medium, having a large number of equi-spaced lines coated with aluminum. Gaps in the grating represent transparent places. Light falling on the transparent areas of gratings gets refracted while those falling on the lines are blocked. As a result light passes through the gratings in thin parallel slices. Desired wavelengths of the spectrum are obtained by rotating the grating near the exit slits. Gratings are now produced by holographic technique.

The exit slit: Light from the monochromator passes through a slit before entering into the cells that contain the sample solution. Though the objective of the monochromator is to produce pure light (light of a single wavelength), the light passing out from the monochromator is not absolutely monochromatic. It is usually a mixture of a narrow range of wavelengths. The resolving power of an instrument is controlled by its slit width settings. An increase in the slit width increases the spectral bandwidth and decreases the monochromaticity.

The cuvette: UV region of spectrophotometry refers to the near UV region, i.e. 200 to 400 nm, where quartz cell is used as a sample holder. The atmosphere (gases constituting the atmosphere) is transparent in this region. Absorption by atmospheric oxygen starts near 200 nm. However, wavelengths lesser than 200 nm, can also be used in UV spectrophotometry with special protection. The region of 185–200 nm can be used through nitrogen flushing (oxygen is not allowed to come in contact with sample) or vacuum spectrophotometry.

Detector: The fraction of light that passes through the solution of absorbing species finally reaches the detector. By comparing the light received from the sample cell with that from the reference cell, detector measures how much light the sample has absorbed. It is difficult to measure the quantum of unabsorbed light directly. In older models of spectrophotometers, a photomultiplier tube is used. A photomultiplier tube basically consists of a photoemissive cathode (a cathode that emits electrons when struck by photons of radiation), several dynodes (which emit several electrons for each electron striking them) and an anode. As the light passing through the solution enters the photomultiplier tube and strikes its cathode, emission of electrons takes place. These electrons are accelerated towards the first dynode (an electrode that causes secondary emission of electrons) causing the emission of several electrons for each incident electron. These electrons are then accelerated towards the successive dynodes in a distinct pattern and more and more electrons are produced. The sequential passage of electron from one dynode to another causes multiplication and on an average $10^6 - 10^7$ electrons are produced from every original photon. Finally, the electrons are collected at the anode. The resulting current is amplified and measured. Photomultipliers are very sensitive to UV and visible radiation but intense light damages them. They are limited to measuring low power radiation.

It is desired that only the monochromatic light passing through the sample should reach the detector and be converted into signal. However, sometimes extra light or light of different wavelength may reach the detector. Stray light arises from scattering and refraction inside the monochromator because of faulty optical surfaces. The effect of stray light is highest near the extremes of the wavelength range like near 200 nm in deuterium lamp. If the stary light is of higher wavelength and is unabsorbed by the sample, the detector shows faulty absorption, which is lesser than its true value.

Photodiodes: The newer models of spectrophotometers usually use photodiodes as detector. Photodiodes are much faster than photomultiplier tubes. They can measure absorption at different wavelengths at a time. Light passing through a polychromator gets dispersed and directed to a diode array that measures the whole spectrum at once. A diode array consists of a series of photodiode detectors positioned side by side on a silicon crystal. The array typically contains 200–1000 elements and the scan cycle is extremely fast (100 ms).

Factors affecting Spectrophotometric Measurements

Solvent: The basic guideline of solvent selection is as follows:

1. At the wavelength of measurement, solvent should not absorb light while the analyte should show strong absorption.
2. The analyte must be completely soluble in the solvent to ensure perfect homogenous distribution. Polar substances are soluble in polar solvents whereas nonpolar substances are soluble in nonpolar solvents. For polar substances, water is considered as the ideal solvent. Above 180 nm, water is transparent at all wavelengths in the UV and visual regions. Sometimes, analytes are sensitive to water and reaction may take place. In such cases, pH of the solvent is adjusted in such a way that only one species is present (ions or molecules).

For nonpolar molecules, organic solvents are used. Organic solvents are not as transparent as water. They may absorb light in the region of 200–220 nm. In double beam spectrophotometer, a reference cell is used and weak absorption by solvent may be compensated this way. But if the solvent absorbs strongly (absorbance above 0.4), it should not be used for measurement. In short, while selecting a solvent, we have to ensure that it does not absorb at the wavelength of measurement. Cyclohexane is a good solvent for nonpolar compounds.

Saturated hydrocarbons are transparent in the near UV region, as they need high energy for excitation. Hence, they can be used as a solvent for lipophilic moieties. Saturated hydrocarbons containing oxygen, nitrogen or sulfur possess nonbonding electrons. They can undergo $n - \sigma^*$ transition, which require low energy for excitation. But they too do not show absorption in the near UV region. Alcohol and ethers absorb at wavelengths shorter than 185 nm and hence, can be used as solvents.

Concentration of the Absorbing Species

If we measure the absorbance of the same solution in the same instrument for a number of times, the results may not be exactly the same. There may be small random fluctuation in result due to a number of causes like variations in the light source intensity as well as detector and amplifier noise. This error is expressed as a percentage of the true concentration.

Suppose, C is the true concentration and C_{obs} is the observed concentration. As the nature of the error is random, C_{obs} can be either higher or lower than the true concentration C.

Error of observation is $\Delta C = |C_{obs} - C|$

$$\%\ \text{Relative error} = \frac{\Delta C \times 100}{C} \qquad \text{(Eq. 9.5)}$$

Note C is in the denominator of the equation, which indicates with the increase of measured concentration, the magnitude of the relative error decreases.

The magnitude of the error mainly depends on the type of detector used. In modern instruments where phototube detectors are used, the relative error is minimum when absorbance is 0.869 or the light transmitted is 13.5%. So, it is customary to have a concentration that gives an absorbance around 0.9 for maximum accuracy. In practice absorbances in the range 0.3 to 1.5 are sufficiently reliable. Hence, concentration and cell pathlengths are adjusted in such a way to keep the absorption within this range. Higher concentration and longer pathlength both increase the value of absorbance.

IMPORTANT APPLICATIONS OF UV SPECTROPHOTOMETRY

1. Structure analysis
2. Quantification

Structure Analysis

Appearance and position of the UV absorption bands can be used for the structure analysis of pharmaceutical substances. Absorption of light occurs due to the chromophores, a term originally used for unsaturated groups of atoms that produce color. However, –ene, –yne and carbonyl groups, which have loosely bounded electrons can also absorb light in the near UV region and are considered as chromophores. Absorption occurs only when the energy of light equals to that required for an electronic transition. Hence, by studying the nature (intensity and frequency) of the absorbed light, we can understand the types of bonds present in an absorbing species. For excitation, σ electrons of the saturated molecules need very high energy which can be provided by extremely short wavelength radiations. Thus, their absorption bands lie in the vacuum ultraviolet region. π-electrons are present in the multiple bonds and are called 'mobile' electrons. Their basic absorption due to $\pi - \pi^*$ transition is in the 180–200 nm region. The third type is n-electrons or non-bonding electrons. The lone pair of O, N and S are nonbonding electrons, which cause low intensity of absorption. The absorption of carbonyl group at around 280 nm is an example.

Some fully saturated groups (auxochromes) when attached to chromophoric system, can bring changes in the absorption spectra. There are two types of auxochromes: coordinatively unsaturated (e.g. $-NH_2-$, $-S-$) that contain lone pair of electron; and coordinatively saturated (e.g. $-NH_3^+$). The saturated type keeps the absorption spectra largely unaffected but they can affect the position of absorption maxima.

The wavelength of maximum absorption is usually selected for measurement of concentration. At λ_{max} noise or the small errors in setting the wavelength scale has minimum effect on the measured absorbance and accuracy of the measurement is maximum. The shift of absorption maxima also indicates the nature of the group attached to a chromophoric system.

Principles involved in the Calculation of λ_{max}

Woodward-Fieser Rules

Robert Burns Woodward and Louis Fieser have derived certain empirical rules with the help of which we can calculate the absorption maxima of a compound in UV spectroscopy from the chromophores present and shifts due to solvents. The formulas are called Woodward-Fieser Rules and differ for a set of chemical classes. Some of these values of various chromophores belonging to major chemical categories like dienes, enone, aromatic compounds acids and its derivatives are given Table 9.1.

In UV spectroscopy, essentially the electrons are excited from ground state to excited state after absorbing the UV radiation. But this transition from ground state to excited state does not depend only on the electron. The nuclei which hold the electrons together in bond formation play an important role. The nuclei determine the strength with which the electrons are bound and thus influence the energy difference between the ground state and the excited states. Therefore, absorption of a characteristic wavelength is characteristic of group of atoms rather than that of electrons. Such group of atoms is called chromophore.

During UV absorption most probable transition in the electrons occurs from highest occupied molecular orbital (HOMO) to lowest unoccupied molecular orbital (LUMO). The energy difference between two states varies from 120–650 KJ/mol. The order of lowest occupied molecular orbital (LOMO) is s then p and then n (nonbonding orbital).

The transition takes place between $\sigma \rightarrow \sigma^*$, $\sigma \rightarrow \pi^*$, $\pi \rightarrow \pi^*$, $n \rightarrow \sigma^*$ or π^*.

The transitions that involve a change in the spin quantum number of the electron during transition are not allowed and are called forbidden transitions, e.g. $n \rightarrow \pi^*$.

1. Woodward-Fieser Rules for Calculating the Diene Compounds

An extension in conjugation of double bond causes a bathochromic shift in the UV spectra and also increases intensity of absorption. This can be attributed to the fact that the presence of conjugated double bonds pushes the electronic energy levels of chromophores together, thus lesser energy is required to produce a transition from an occupied molecular to unoccupied molecular orbital, hence, the wavelength becomes longer.

Aliphatic dienes can be classified as cisoid or transoid. The values for this class of compounds are given in Table 9.1.

Table 9.1: Woodward-Fieser rules for dienes

Base value for heteroannular diene (transoid)/acyclic diene	214 nm
Base value for homoannular diene (cisoid)	253
Aliphatic	
Transoid	217
Cisoid	245
Increments	
Homocyclic diene	+39
Double bond extending conjugation	+30
Alkyl substituent or ring residue	+5
Exocyclic double bond	+5
Acetate group	+0
Ether group	+6
Thioether group	+30
Bromine, chlorine	+5
Tertiary amine group	+30

Exocyclic double bonds are the double bonds which are in *conjugation* but present in different ring.

Ring residue are the single bonds or the alkyl groups attached directly to the double bonds (ring residue in the above example is shown as the line cutting the single bonds).

Double bond extending conjugation is the number of double bonds which are in conjugation with the basic diene (chromophore) system.

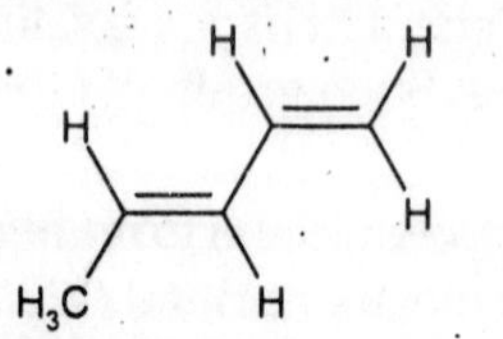

Acyclic diene	214
Alkyl group	5
	219

Observed value = 220 nm

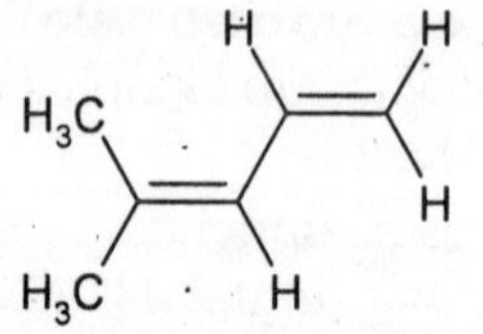

Acyclic diene	214
Alkyl group (2 × 5)	10
	224

Observed value = 225 nm

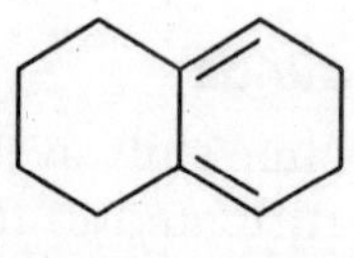

Homoannular diene (cisoid)
λ value = 253

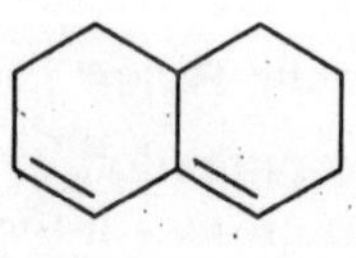

Heteroannular diene (transoid)
λ value = 214

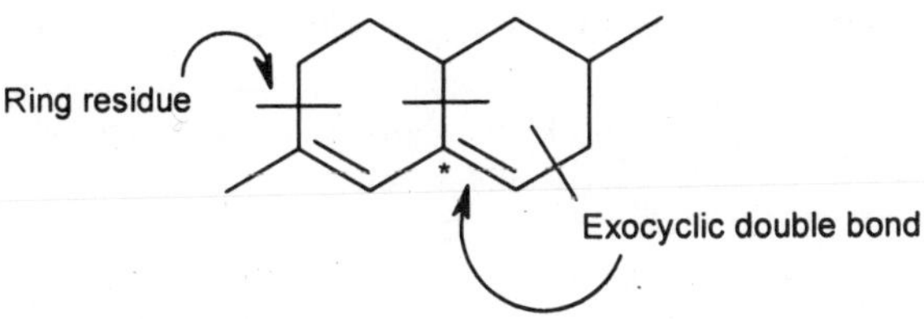

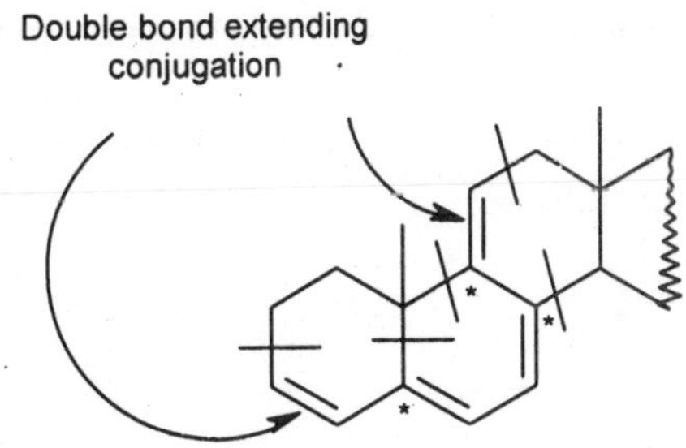

Transoid	214
Ring residue (3 × 5)	15
Exocyclic double bond	5
Alkyl substituent	5
	239

Observed = 240 nm

Cisoid	253
Ring residue (5 × 5)	25
Exocyclic double bond (3 × 5)	15
Double bond extending conjugation (2 × 30)	60
	353

Observed= 355 nm

2. Woodward-Fieser Rules for Calculating Enones (Table 9.2)

A double bond in conjugation with a carbonyl group leads to intense absorption, because of transition of electrons from $\pi \rightarrow \pi^*$ in carbonyl group.

Table 9.2: Woodward-Fieser rules for enone absorption

Core chromophore		*Substituent and influence*	
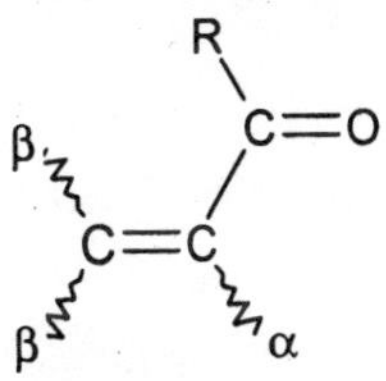	R = Alkyl 215 nm R = H 210 nm R = OR′ 195 nm	*α-*	*Substituents*
		R-(Alkyl group)	+10 nm
		Cl-(Chloro group)	+15
		Br-(Chloro group)	+25
		HO-(Hydroxyl group)	+35
		RO-(Alkoxyl group)	+35
		RCO_2-(Acyl group)	+6
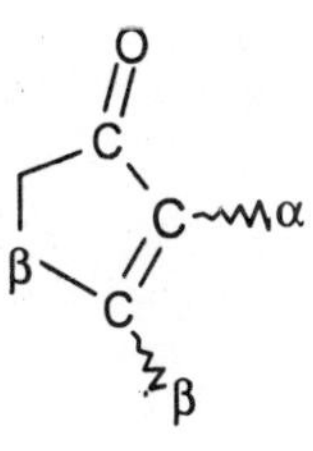	Cyclopentenone 202 nm	*β-*	*Substituents*
		R-(Alkyl group)	+12 nm
		Cl-(Chloro group)	+12
		Br-(Chloro group)	+30
		HO-(Hydroxyl group)	+30
		RO-(Alkoxyl group)	+30
		RCO_2-(Acyl group)	+6
		RS-(Sulfide group)	+85
		R_2N-(Amino group)	+95
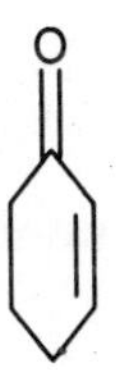	Six-membered enone ring 215 nm	*α and β-*	*Substituents*
		R-(Alkyl group)	+18 nm
		HO-(Hydroxyl group)	+50 nm
		RO-(Alkoxyl group)	+30 nm

(Contd.)

Table 9.2: Woodward-Fieser rules for enone absorption *(Contd.)*

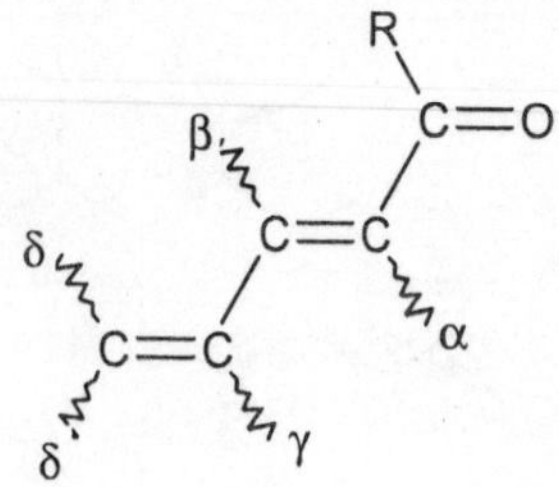

Further δ-Conjugation	
C = C (Double bond) ...	+30
C_6H_5 (Phenyl group) ...	+60
General	
Acyclic dienone	245 nm
Homocyclic diene	+39
Double bond extending conjugation	+30
α-ring residue	+10
β-ring residue	+12
δ-ring residue	+18
Exocyclic double bond adds	+5 nm
Solvent correction:	
Water = +8;	
Methanol/ethanol = 0;	
Ether = +7;	
Hexane/cyclohexane = +11	

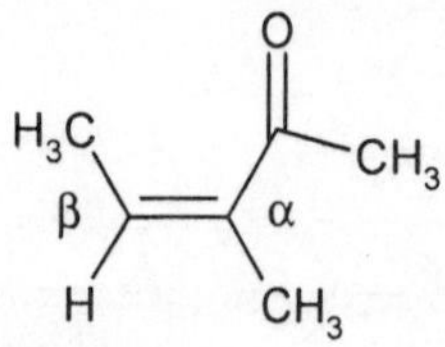

Acyclic enone	215
α-CH_3	10
β-CH_3	12
	237

Observed = 240 nm

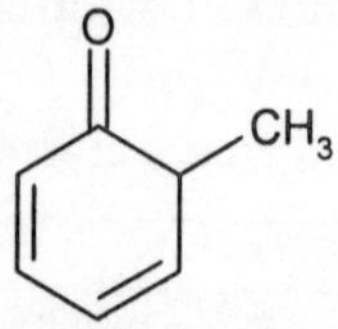

Six-membered enone	215
Double bond extending conjugation	30
δ-ring residue	18
Homocyclic diene	39
	302

Observed = 300 nm

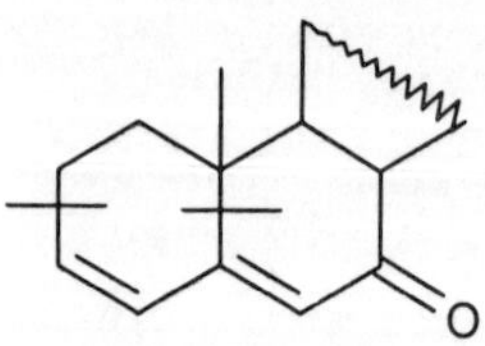

Six-membered enone	215
Double bond extending conjugation	30
Exocyclic double bond	5
β-ring residue	12
δ-ring residue	18
	280

Observed = 280 nm

3. Woodward-Fieser Rules for Calculating the Conjugated Carbonyl Compounds (Table 9.3)

Aldehydes, esters and carboxylic acids have different base values than ketones.

Table 9.3: Woodward-Fieser rules for conjugated carbonyl compound absorption

Unsaturated system	*Base value*
Aldehyde	208
With α or β alkyl groups	220
With α, β or β, β alkyl groups	230
With α, β, β alkyl groups	242
Acid or ester	
With α or β alkyl groups	208
With α, β or β, β alkyl groups	217
Group value–exocyclic α, β double bond	+5
Group value–endocyclic α, β bond in 5- or 7-membered ring	+5
Solvent correction	*Increment*
Water	+8
Ethanol, methanol	0
Chloroform	−1
Dioxane	−5
Ether	−7
Hydrocarbon	−11

4. Woodward-Fieser Rules for Aromatic Compounds (Table 9.4)

Table 9.4: Woodward-Fieser rules for aromatic compounds with various substitutions

	Substituent in the aromatic ring	*Primary peak*		*Secondary peak*	
		λ_{max}	ε	λ_{max}	ε
Electron donating	−H	203.5	7,400	254	204
	$-CH_3$	207	7,000	261	225
	−Cl	210	7,400	264	190
	−Br	210	7,900	261	192
	−OH	211	6,200	270	1,450
	−O−	235	9,400	287	2,600
	$-OCH_3$	217	6,400	269	1,480
	$-NH_2$	230	8,600	280	1,430
	$-NH_3+$	203	7,500	254	169
Electron withdrawing	CN	224	13,000	271	1,000
	−C (O) OH	230	11,600	273	970
	−C (O) O−	224	8,700	268	560
	−C (O) H−	250	11,400		
	$-C (O) CH_3$	224	9,800		
	$-NO_2$	269	7,800		

Quantitative Determination by UV Spectroscopy

UV spectrophotometry is widely used for purpose of quantification of drugs. The procedure is simple. A solution of the absorbing species is made in a transparent solvent. The absorbance of this solution is measured at different wavelengths. However, the exact procedure involved depends upon the nature and purity of the samples.

Determination of Concentration from a given Absorptivity Value

For certain compounds the absorptivity value is given in official books. The molar absorptivity is recorded for pure substances and unknown concentration of such substances can be determined from these reference values. However, this method is not applicable for the majority of the substances. Variation in the sensitivity of instrument, variability of sample handling cause deviation from the standard. Hence, only stable drugs with broad absorption bands, unaffected by the instrumental variation can be determined by this method. The method is particularly useful where reference drugs are expensive and difficult to obtain.

Example 1: Suppose, the absorbance of drug solution was found to be 0.5 at 241 nm. The A (1%, 1 cm) of the drug is reported to be 550 at λ_{max} (241 nm). Calculate the concentration of the unknown solution.

According to the Beer-Lambert's law,

$$\text{Absorbance} = A^{1\%}_{1\,\text{cm}} \times b \times c$$

Since the pathlength is 1 cm, $b = 1$

$$\therefore \quad 0.5 = 550 \times 1 \times c$$

$$\therefore \quad c = 0.5 \div 550\%$$

$$c = 0.000909 \text{ gm/100 ml.}$$

Note as $A^{1\%}_{1\,\text{cm}}$ means the concentration of the drug is 1 gm in 100 ml solution, the units of unknown concentration is also expressed in gm/100 ml or percentage.

1. *Determination of the unknown concentration from the calibration curves:*

Calibration curves are necessary when it is essential to confirm the proportionality of absorbance as function of concentration. It is most relevant in colorimetry or visible spectrophotometry where colorless substances are converted to colored derivatives by reaction in which incomplete reaction may result in erroneous result and lack of linearity. Calibration curve is constructed in such cases to validate the process and confirm linearity. In pharmaceutical research, this method is routinely used for the determination of drug release from experimental formulations.

Typically, 4–6 standard solutions of different concentrations are prepared. Prior knowledge of absorptivity helps in selection of concentrations. Solutions are usually made in such a way as to have the absorbance ranging from 0.1 to 0.9. Absorbances of the standard solutions are plotted against concentration to draw a straight line. A regression analysis is also carried to establish the quantitative relationship between concentration and absorbance, treating the standard concentrations as independent variables and absorbances as dependent variables. Once the relationship is established, unknown concentrations can be determined by substituting the value of absorbance in the equation.

Example 2: Construct a standard curve from the given concentration–absorbance data.

Conc (μg/ml)	*Absorbance*
00	0.002
10	0.15
20	0.30
30	0.44
40	0.58
50	0.75

The regression analysis of the concentration–absorbance data yields the equation $Y = 0.014X + 0.0001$, where Y represents absorbance and X, the concentration. The value of the intercept is 0.0001. Ideally the intercept should be 0. Sometimes, regression analysis yields real intercepts. In those cases, test of intercept should be carried out (see the test of intercept in Chapter 3). The null hypothesis for intercept is stated as H_0: $A = 0$.

If the null hypothesis is accepted, it indicates the intercept has resulted from the random error of measurement and intercept is considered insignificant. If rejected the intercept should be considered in calculation of the concentration. Often a repeated experiment (determination of absorbance twice or thrice and taking the average value) increases the accuracy of the calibration curve.

2. *Simultaneous estimation of two or more analytes*

Occasionally, we come across situations where sample to be measured contains more than one analyte. Assay of the multi-drug formulations is an example and simultaneous estimation method can be used for estimating such samples. The process involves determination of absorbance of the sample mixture at more than one wavelength.

If a sample contains two absorbing species X and Y and both absorb at the λ_{max} of the other, they can be estimated without prior separation in the following manner.

Choice of Wavelengths

X and Y are prepared at equimolar concentrations and absorption spectra are recorded. The wavelengths at which the ratio of absorbance of X and Y are maximum are chosen for the analysis of mixture.

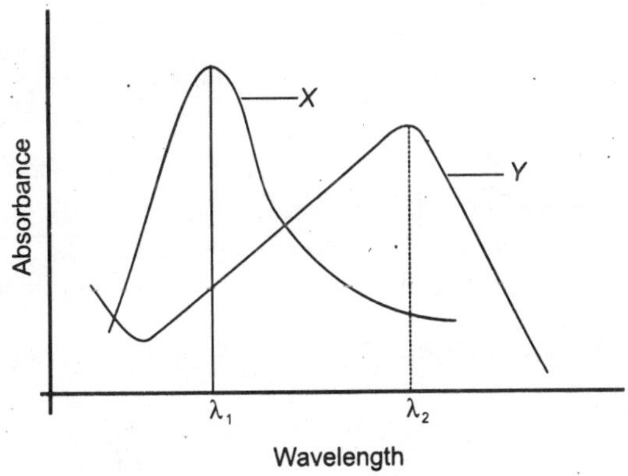

Fig. 9.4: Absorption spectra of X and Y

In Fig. 9.4, ratio of the absorbances X/Y is maximum at λ_1 and that of Y/X is maximum at λ_2. Hence, these two wavelengths should be chosen for analysis.

Developing the Equation

If the molar absorptivity is known, equations can be developed using absorptivity values. Alternatively, calibration curves for both the drugs should be constructed at both the wavelengths and the slope of the regression line can be used to develop the equation.

Let us assume, the recorded λ_{max} of the two analytes X, Y are λ_1 and λ_2.

So molar absorptivities of the drug X at λ_1 and λ_2 are defined as aX_1 and aX_2.

Similarly, molar absorptivities of the drug Y at λ_1 and λ_2 are A_1 and A_2.

The absorbance of the sample mixture (X and Y) at λ_1 and λ_2 are A_1 and A_2.

Absorbance of a sample is denoted by A

$$A = abc$$

Where, a = molar absorptivity, b = cell pathlength and c represents concentration. If the concentration of the analyte X and Y in the mixture is represented as C_x and C_y, absorbance at λ_1 due to X will be aX_1bC_x and that of Y will be aY_1bC_y.

The absorbance of a mixture X and Y at any wavelength is the sum total of their individual absorptions.

The total absorbance is $A_1 = aX_1bC_x + aY_1bC_y$ (Eq. 9.6)

Similarly, $A_2 = aX_1bC_x + aY_1bC_y$ (Eq. 9.7)

Assuming the cell pathlength, i.e. b as 1 cm, and rearranging the Eq. 9.7 we get,

$$C_x = \frac{A_2 - aY_2C_y}{aX_2}$$

Substituting the value of C_x in Eq. 9.6.

$$A_1 = aX_1\left(\frac{A_2 - aY_2C_y}{aX_2}\right) + aY_1C_y$$

$$\therefore \quad A_1aX_2 = A_2aX_1 - aX_1aY_2C_y + aX_2aY_1C_y$$

$$\therefore \quad C_y = \frac{A_1\,aX_2 - A_2\,aX_1}{aX_2\,aY_1 - aX_1aY_2}$$

Similarly, the concentration of X in the sample is,

$$C_x = \frac{A_2\,aY_1 - A_1\,aY_2}{aX_2\,aY_1 - aX_1aY_2}$$

Simultaneous Equation using a Calibration Curve

When a mixture contains two or more drugs and we do not have the molar absorptivity value, calibration curves can be used to determine their concentration.

Example 3: The λ_{max} of two drugs A and B are 222 and 242 nm respectively. Given are the data tables showing their absorbance at various concentrations. Develop an equation for determining the concentration of individual drugs in the mixture of these two drugs.

The optical density of A at various concentration levels at 222 and 242 nm.

Concentration of A (mg/ml)	*OD at 222 nm*	*OD at 242 nm*
0	0	0
4	0.223	0.011
8	0.405	0.019
12	0.559	0.023
16	0.739	0.028
20	0.895	0.035

The optical density of B at various concentration levels at 222 and 242 nm

Concentration of B (mg/ml)	*OD at 222 nm*	*OD at 242 nm*
0	0	0
2	0.101	0.172
4	0.186	0.313
6	0.253	0.415
8	0.342	0.563
10	0.396	0.691

Let us use the symbol X to indicate concentration of A and Y to indicate concentration of B. First, regression equations are to be constructed at both the wavelengths.

If the OD represents optical density, the calibration curve for A at 222 nm can be written as,

$OD = 0.046X$ and that at 242 nm is $OD = 0.0018X$ respectively.

For B the relationships at 222 and 242 nm are and $OD = 0.041Y$ and $OD = 0.071Y$ respectively.

When two drugs are present in solution, both absorb at both the wavelengths and absorbance recorded is sum total of the individual absorbances.

$$\text{At 222 nm } OD_1 = 0.046X + 0.041Y \qquad \text{(Eq. 9.8)}$$

$$\text{At 242 nm } OD_2 = 0.0018X + 0.071Y \qquad \text{(Eq. 9.9)}$$

Where,

X = concentration of A

Y = concentration of B.

OD_1 = absorbance of the mixture at 222 nm

OD_2 = absorbance of the mixture at 242 nm

To cancel the value of Y from the equation, Eq. 9.8 is multiplied by 1.73,

$$0.079X + 0.071Y = OD_1 \times 1.73 \qquad \text{(Eq. 9.10)}$$

$$0.0018X + 0.071Y = OD_2 \qquad \text{(Eq. 9.9)}$$

Subtracting Eq. 9.9 from Eq. 9.10.

We get,

$$X = \frac{OD_1 \times 1.73 - OD_2}{0.0772}$$

$$X = \text{concentration of } A$$

Similarly, by multiplying Eq. 9.9 with 25.66 we get,

$$0.046X + 1.82Y = OD_2 \times 25.66 \text{ (Eq. 9.11)}$$

Subtracting Eq. 9.8 from Eq. 9.11

$$Y = \frac{OD_2 \times 25.66 - OD_1}{1.78}$$

Derivative Spectroscopy

Sometimes, samples may contain impurities and cause irrelevant absorption and insert error into the drug assay. In the derivative spectroscopy, instead of normal absorbance, the first or higher derivative of absorbance is recorded with respect to the wavelength. For this, the normal or a zero order spectrum has to be converted to first, second or higher order spectra. An ideal zero order absorption band is Gaussian in nature. The first derivative spectrum is a plot of the rate of change of absorption with wavelength

$$\left(\frac{dA}{d\lambda}\right) \text{ against the wavelength.}$$

The maximum positive and maximum negative slope of the normal spectra gets the position of maxima and minima in the derivative curve.

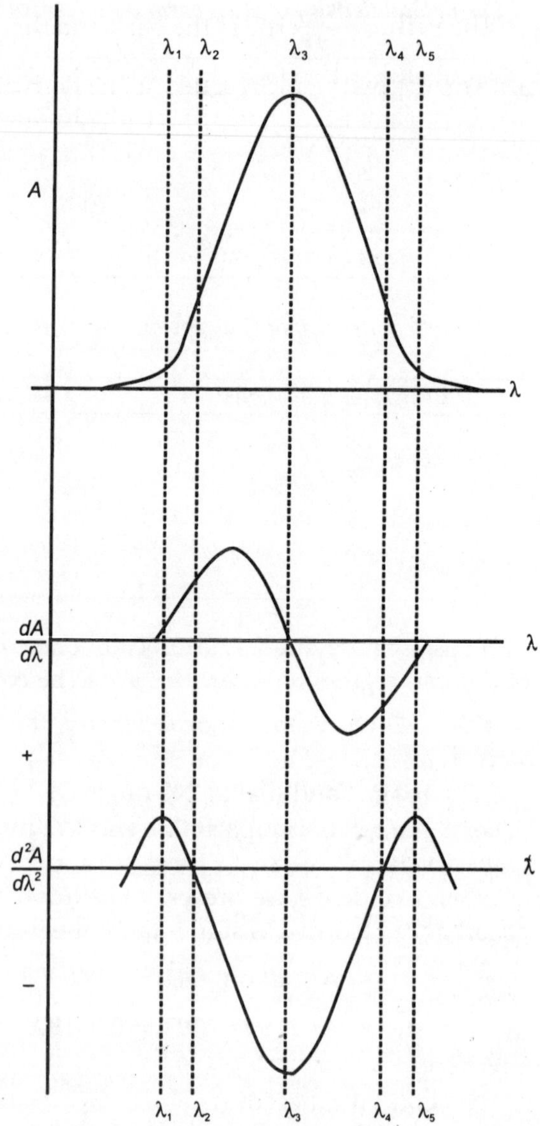

Fig. 9.5: The normal (A), first $\left(\frac{dA}{d\lambda}\right)$ and second derivative $\left(\frac{d^2A}{d\lambda^2}\right)$ spectra of a compound

To clarify the idea let us take the absorption spectra of a substance X. Two wavelengths λ_1, λ_2 are on the left side of the peak and two wavelengths λ_4, λ_5 are on the right side of the peak whereas λ_3 is the wavelength of peak absorption (Fig. 9.5).

In the given figure (A), the maximum positive slope, is on the left side and the maximum negative slope is on the right side of the peak. Consequently, the peak and trough of the first derivative spectra have occurred at these points.

The value of $\frac{dA}{d\lambda}$ is 0 at the peak and the first derivative graph also shows λ_3 as the crossover point. Simply stated, a first derivative spectrum is characterized by a maxima, a minima and a crossover point which coincides with the λ_{max} of the normal spectrum. The second derivative spectrum is characterized by two maxima and an inverted band the minimum of which corresponds to the λ_{max} of the normal spectra.

Conversion of normal spectra into derivative spectra has several advantages. An even order spectrum is of narrower bandwidth than its zero order spectrum.

Provided Beer's law is obeyed in the fundamental region, amplitudes of derivative spectra are proportional to the concentration of the analytes. It is known that $A = abc$ and is conventionally expressed as,

$$A = \varepsilon c l$$

$$\therefore \quad \frac{dA}{d\lambda} = \frac{d\varepsilon}{d\lambda} cl \qquad \text{(Eq. 9.12)}$$

For second derivative,

$$\therefore \quad \frac{d^2A}{d\lambda^2} = \frac{d^2\varepsilon}{d\lambda^2} cl \qquad \text{(Eq. 9.13)}$$

Derivative spectrum shows better resolution of overlapping bands. The distance from the minimum to maximum is inversely proportional to the spectral bandwidth raised to the power of derivative order.

$$D \propto \left(\frac{1}{W}\right)^n \qquad \text{(Eq. 9.14)}$$

This allows selective determination of the absorbing species in presence of interfering substances. The largest amplitude unaffected by other bands is to be measured for quantification. For quantitative purpose, second and fourth derivatives are the most frequently employed derivative orders (Fig. 9.6).

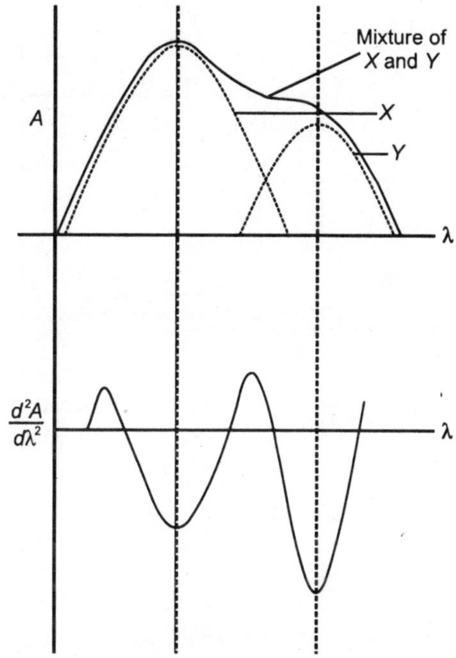

Fig. 9.6: The spectra of mixture of two drugs *X* and *Y* and the second derivative spectrum of the mixture showing resolution into individual bands

In the derivative spectrum, the ability to detect and measure minor spectral features is considerably enhanced. This enhancement of characteristic spectra details can distinguish between very similar spectra and follow subtle change in a spectrum. Moreover, it can be used in quantitative analysis to measure the concentration of an analyte, whose peak is obscured by a larger overlapping peak due to the presence of molecules other than the analyte in the sample. Widespread availability of HPLC has reduced the use of derivative spectra for this purpose but it is still useful for detecting the presence of contaminants in a sample. Compounds synthesized in the laboratory often contain traces of reagents that absorb almost at the same wavelengths as that of main compound. Such contamination can be detected by this process.

Two spectra are shown in the Fig. 9.7. The graph on the left hand side shows the normal and first derivative spectra of a pure analyte. Normal peak is well defined. So are the peaks in first derivative spectra, indicating the absence of contaminants.

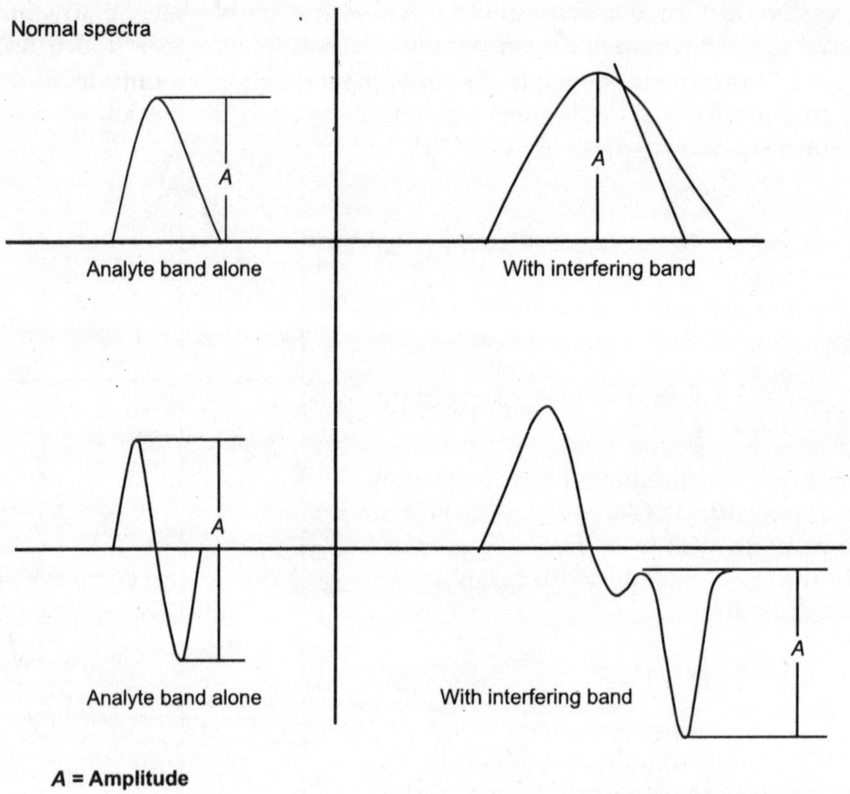

Fig. 9.7: Comparison of zero and first derivative spectrum left side with analyte bands alone, right side with interfering bands

The spectrum on the right hand side is not clearly defined. The peak is not sharp. It is wide resulting from an interfering band. Conventionally, the natural bandwidth is measured at half peak height and peaks are more or less symmetrical. However, the right half of the spectra with interfering substances is broader than the left half indicating absorbance by more than one molecule. In such cases, it is advantageous to base the measurement on the derivative spectra. Referring to the derivative spectra in the lower right of figure, it is easier to take the measure of the analyte intensity as the vertical distance between the adjacent maximum and minimum of the first derivative if the interfering band is at least a factor of 2 broader than the analyte band.

A variety of different experimental techniques have been used to obtain derivative spectra. If the spectrum has been recorded digitally or is otherwise available in computer readable form, the differentiation can be done numerically. Alternatively, the derivative spectra may be recorded directly in real time, either by wavelength modulation or by obtaining the time derivative of the spectrum scanned at a constant rate. In the latter case, a quite simple electronic differentiator can be used. Several commercial spectrometers capable of recording derivative spectra are now available. Dual-wavelength spectrometers can obtain first derivative spectra by wavelength modulation.

BIBLIOGRAPHY

1. AH Beckett and JB Stenlake, *Practical Pharmaceutical Chemistry* (eds) CBS Publishers, Ist Indian edition 1997.
2. DG Watson, *Pharmaceutical Analysis*, 2nd ed, Elsevier Limited, 2005.
3. Michael Thomas, Ultraviolet and visible spectroscopy in analytical chemistry open learning series, John Wiley and Sons, 1996.
4. Willard et al, *Instrumental Method of Analysis*, CBS Publishers & Distributors, 6th ed., Delhi, 1996, http://teaching.shu.ac.uk/hwb/chemistry/tutorials/molspec/uvvisab3.htm.

10 High Performance Liquid Chromatography

INTRODUCTION

High performance liquid chromatography (HPLC) is a versatile tool widely used in the routine analysis of pharmaceutical substances in the industries as well as for research purpose. HPLC is a sophisticated technique where the samples are simultaneously separated and quantified. In pharmaceutical research, quantity of the synthesized compounds is often small and they contain trace amount of source compounds. So, before quantification, we need to clean the samples of these trace materials. Though there are many techniques for separation, few are as efficient as HPLC. HPLC does the dual job of separation and quantification at great speed. The technique is popular due to its high sensitivity (can detect and quantify substances at the microgram and nanogram levels) and its efficacy to analyze multi-component real life samples. As a preparative technique, it allows quantitative recovery of many labile substances from milligram to kilogram levels. Majority of the existing components can be separated and quantified by this technique. It is almost indispensable for the analysis of drugs in biological samples like blood and tissue fluids. This chapter introduces the basic concepts of HPLC separation with special emphasis on reverse phase HPLC, which is extensively used in pharmaceutical industries.

Applications of HPLC in Pharmacy

Drug discovery: To isolate and identify the lead compounds in drug development research.

Pharmaceutical development: To develop dosage forms with optimized delivery and stability profiles.

Pharmacokinetic studies: For evaluation of metabolic and pharmacokinetic profiles in animal and human clinical trials.

Quality control: For assessment of manufactured dosage forms with respect to dose strength and drug release.

Limitations of the Technique

Though HPLC has many advantages, it has a few limitations too. HPLC does not have a universal detector. So even if a sample is separated into its constituents by the column, all the components may not be measured or identified by a single detector. Detector should be chosen according to the nature of the analytes. Moreover, HPLC instruments are complex machines, which require skilled operators.

BASIC CONCEPTS

The basic concept of HPLC separation is quite simple. It is the same as any other chromatography technique like solid and gas chromatography, where individual components of a mixture are retarded by a stationary phase at differential rates. The degree of retention or retardation depends upon the analyte's molecular affinity for the stationary phase. However, HPLC has a significant difference too. While in other chromatography techniques, stationary phase is solid, HPLC has a liquid like stationary phase. Choice of column, which contains the stationary phase, depends on the nature of sample to be assayed. For good separation, the analytes should have good affinity for the stationary phase, which helps to slow down their movement through the column. The most common stationary phase used in pharmacy is bonded porous silica, packed in a column.

The mobile phase (flowing liquid) can be an organic solvent or a mixture of aqueous and organic solvents. The polarity of mobile phase can be adjusted to a desired value by using combination of solvents. Many modern HPLC use small particle columns, which allow tight packing. Solvents while passing through the column experience high resistance. For overcoming this resistance to flow, mobile phase is pumped at high pressure.

Mechanism of Separation within the Column

A sequence of events takes place within the column during chromatography. The process is analogous to the solvent extraction process. In solvent extraction, mixtures of components are dissolved in a solvent and shaken with another immiscible solvent. Due to shaking mixing takes place and some of the solutes from the original solvent get transferred into the new solvent. The fraction transferred depends on the affinity of the solute for the new solvent. If the affinity of the analyte is higher for the new solvent (e.g. 2 times that of the original solvent) partition coefficient of the substance (new/old solvent) will be 2. The amount transferred in the new solvent will be determined by this partition coefficient. If equilibrium is attained, the ratio of the solute concentrations in new solvent will be twice that of the original solvent. However, once the extracting solvent is poured off and some fresh extracting solvent is added, a new equilibrium is established and more solutes are transferred into the fresh solvent. In HPLC, mobile phase is the solvent that extracts solutes from the stationary phase. Each of the extraction steps can be compared with one theoretical plate. Within the chromatographic column too, analytes, which have greater affinity for extracting solvent (mobile phase), get transferred fast and come out of the column faster than the ones more strongly bonded to the stationary phase. The passage of a solute through the HPLC column can be visualized from Fig. 10.1.

Let us assume 100 microgram of an analyte is injected into the column and its affinity for the stationary and mobile phase is same (partition coefficient 1). After injecting into the column, the entire quantity is located at the first theoretical plate. As mobile phase flows over that plate, the analyte gets distributed between the two phases equally. So out of 100 microgram, 50 microgram gets transferred to the mobile phase and the rest 50 microgram is retained by the stationary phase. As this mobile phase carrying the analyte moves forward, it comes in contact with the stationary phase of the second plate. Here again, half of the analyte is transferred to the stationary phase. This process of transfer between stationary and mobile phase continues throughout the column.

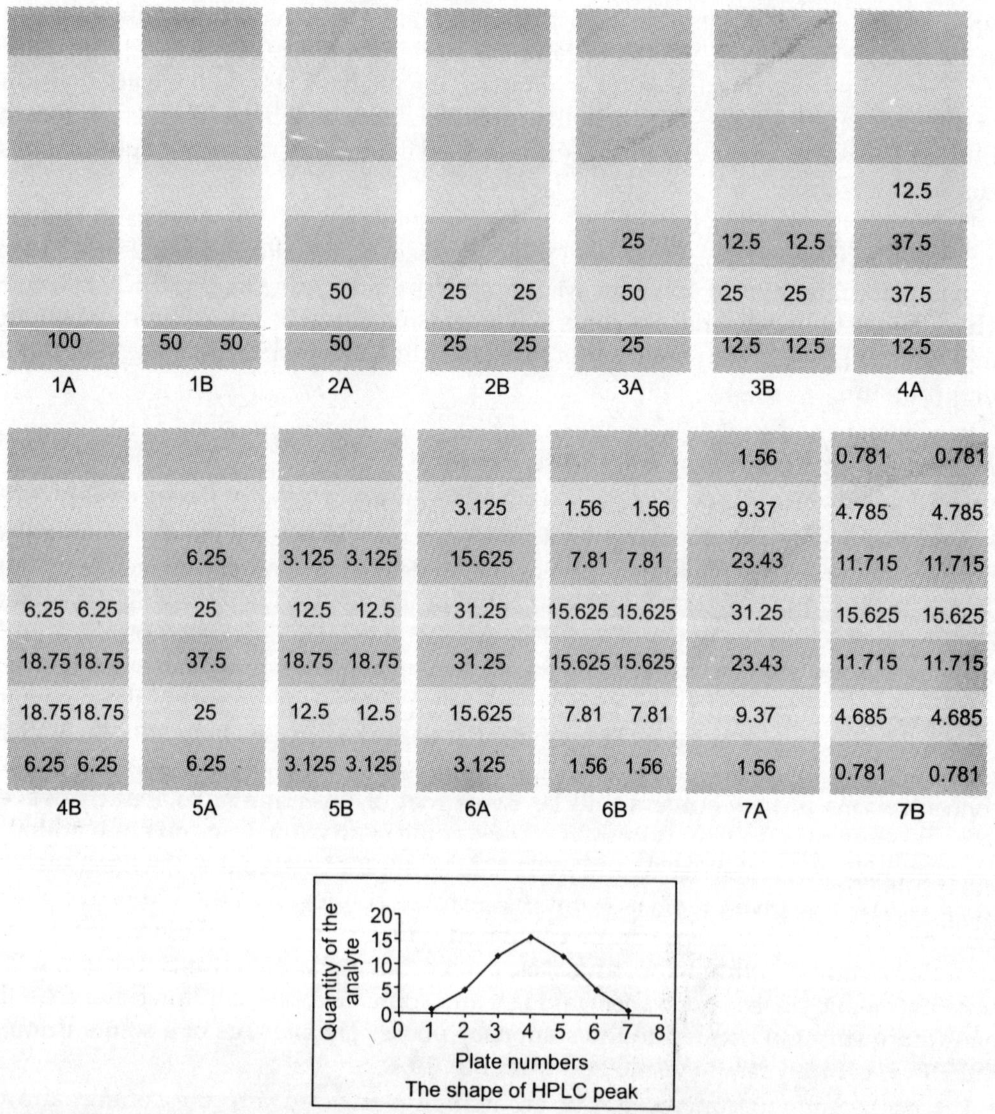

Fig. 10.1: Schematic presentation of analytes in different plates during chromatography

If the quantity of the solute present at different plates at a given time is plotted against plate number, we can see a Gaussian distribution.

1.A. Immediately after injection.

1.B. Solute distributed between stationary and mobile phase (1st plate).

2.A. Mobile phase has reached the 2nd plate.

2.B. Equilibrium has established. In the 1st plate, fresh mobile phase has drawn more solute. In the 2nd plate, mobile phase has donated solute to the stationary phase.

3.A. Mobile phase from 2nd plate has reached 3rd plate after losing half of its analyte content to the stationary phase of 2nd plate. The total content in the 2nd plate is the highest as it is enriched by mobile phase from the first plate, which has carried analyte from the 1st plate.

3.B. No net transfer of the analyte in the 2nd plate as concentrations are same in both the phases.

4.A. Mobile phase from 3rd plate has reached the 4th plate.

4.B. Equilibrium is established again. Note that, the 1st plate has lost more solute to the fresh solvent.

5.A. Mobile phase from 4th plate has reached the 5th plate.

5.B. Equilibrium established.

6.A & B. Note that 3rd and 4th plates have the highest content.

7.A. Note that the highest quantity (peak) is right at the middle (4th plate) and the 1st plate is almost exhausted.

If the solute has higher affinity for the extracting solvent (partition coefficient > 1), the elution band will have sharp peak and if less than 1, the band will look a bit flat.

Suppose, a mixture having three components *X*, *Y*, *Z* is to be separated. Of the three components, *X* has the highest affinity for the column packing and *Y*, the lowest. While moving through the column *X* will be the most retarded (because of its affinity) and *Y*, the least retarded. So within the column, *Y* will travel faster than other components and reach the detector first. If all three components have similar detection properties, e.g. light absorption, they can be detected by the same detector. Hence, these components can be detected as well as quantified in a single step only.

Figure 10.2 shows the absorption bands of *X*, *Y* and *Z* at different timings. Initially all the components are close to one another. The flow of mobile phase drives them forward and as they move through the column, the components with less affinity for the stationary phase (*Y* and *Z*) move faster than *X*, which is strongly bonded to column packing. Hence, *X*, elutes last. The figure shows the absorption band for *Y* appearing first and for *X* the last.

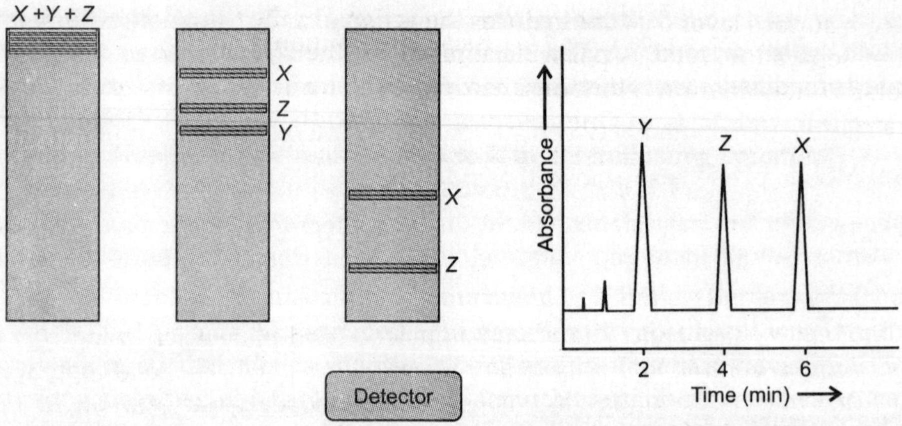

Fig. 10.2: Order of elution in reverse phase chromatography (The most hydrophilic molecule is eluted first)

In HPLC with UV detectors, the area of the absorption bands recorded by the detector is related to the concentration profiles of substances whereas time of appearance of such bands identifies its type.

End-capping

The actual mechanism of separation in HPLC is differential partitioning. The column is packed with fine particles, which acts as a support for the stationary phase. Recently polymers (e.g. polyethers, poly methacrylates, etc.) and hybrid materials have been introduced but support materials are mostly silica-based. Though silica (SiO_2) is the dominant support material, it is rarely used as such. On the surface of silica, exist the silanol groups, which are strongly adsorptive in nature. The silanol groups (Si-OH) are bonded with monochlorosilanes to create a hydrophobic 'liquid-like' stationary phase. However, due to steric hindrance, neutralization of all the silanols is not possible. Presence of free silanol may reduce the efficiency of separation by adsorbing one or more constituents of the sample. Unreacted silanols remaining after the bonding step are further reacted with smaller silanes to reduce the absorptive properties. The process is called end-capping (Fig. 10.3).

Different Modes of HPLC

HPLC techniques used in pharmaceutical analysis can be categorized into four major separation modes; normal phase chromatography, reversed phase chromatography, ion exchange chromatography and size exclusion chromatography (Fig. 10.4).

Normal Phase Chromatography (NPC)

It uses a polar stationary phase. In this, polar analytes get adsorbed and move slowly through the column due to strong interactions with the silanol groups. Initially, the free surface silanol groups of silica were widely used for this purpose. But now, it is believed a surface layer of water reduces the activity of the silanol group and results in better separation. NPC is particularly used for the cleaning up of samples from nonpolar contamination. Nonpolar components are not retarded in this type of separation and elute fast. One disadvantage of this mode of separation is the contamination of the polar surfaces by the sample components. Hence, modern NPC columns have polar functional groups (e.g. amino or cyano groups) bonded to the silanol groups.

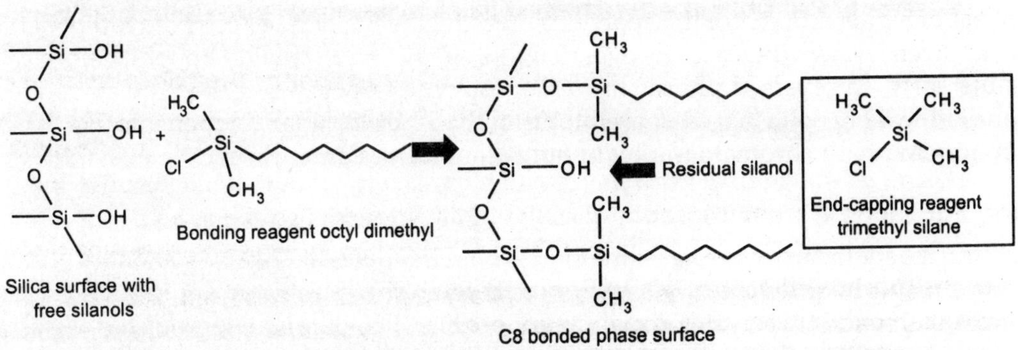

Fig. 10.3: Concept of end-capping

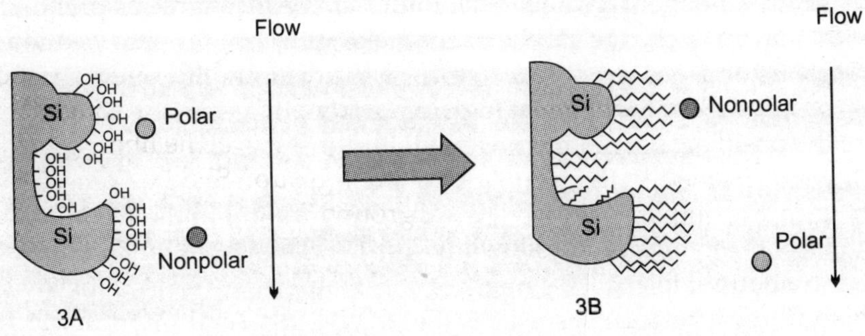

3A. The stationary phase has affinity for polar molecules (normal phase).
3B. The –OH group is replaced by octyl dimethyl silane and it shows affinity for nonpolar molecules (reverse phase).

Fig. 10.4: Stationary phase of normal and reversed phase chromatography

Reversed Phase Chromatography (RPC)

To exert a therapeutic effect, drug substances must cross the tissue and cell barriers, which are lipophilic in nature. Hence, most of pharmaceuticals have got some degree of lipophilicity and are suitable for reversed phase chromatography in which stationary phases are lipophilic in nature. In RPC, the silanol groups (Si-OH) of the silica support are bonded with monochlorosilanes to create a hydrophobic 'liquid-like' stationary phase. While flowing through the column, components get partitioned into these bonded layers and substances of higher lipophilicity get more retarded compared to the ones of lower lipophilicity and elute later. Hence, the lipophilic compounds are eluted late and polar constituents elute fast. However, there is no specific time for a particular substance to elute from the column. The time of elution largely depends upon the nature of mobile phase, which carry the analytes within the column. The residence time of a component can be increased in a column by using a mobile phase, which has low affinity for the analyte. Similarly, retention time can be reduced by using a mobile phase of higher affinity for the analyte. Increasing the fraction of lipophilic components in a solvent system increases its overall lipophilicity and a strongly lipophilic drug can elute early. In reversed phase chromatography, irrespective of the type of bonded phase, the more polar ingredients elute faster than the less polar components (Fig. 10.2). In normal phase chromatography lipophilic molecules elute earlier.

Ion Exchange Chromatography (IEC)

In IEC, the stationary phase has some ionic groups bonded to it. Typical stationary phases contain sulphonate (cation exchange) and quaternary ammonium groups (anion exchange) bonded to polymeric or silica support (Fig. 10.5). Sulphonate group has negative charge but its counter ions are positive, e.g. Na^+. The counterions are loosely bound and can be exchanged with the similarly charged analytes. When a sample is injected into the ion exchange column, positive ions get attached to negative ions of the stationary phase and negative ions get attached to the stationary positive groups. Hence, a moving analyte with a positive charge can be exchanged with the stationary counter ions of sulphonate group and get temporarily stuck in the column. But when a mobile phase containing positively charged ions at high ionic strength passes through the column, it can replace the positive analyte from its binding site. But as the liberated analyte flows forward, it gets attached to the next sulphonate group. Since this process continues repeatedly with the numerous sulphonate groups throughout the column, the overall migration rate of the ionic moiety slows down and it elutes from the column much later compared to a neutral moiety. This mode of chromatography is used for separation of biologicals and ionic substances, especially the amino acids. As amino acids do not absorb strongly in UV or visible region, it is made to undergo a reaction to form color derivatives, which can be detected at 550 nm. However, as the concentration of the ions can be easily measured by conductivity change, IEC systems often come with a conductivity detector.

Size Exclusion Chromatography (SEC)

As the name indicates molecular size of an analyte is the main criterion for separation in this type of chromatography. Usually, the column is packed with cross-linked polystyrene beads of controlled pore size. In a heterogeneous sample, which contains molecules of various sizes, the smaller particles get trapped into the pores whereas the larger ones are excluded. Solvents like toluene or tetrahydrofuran are used as mobile phases to elute this type of columns. In this, high molecular weight molecules elute faster and the elution band shows a gradual decrease in molecular weights. Use

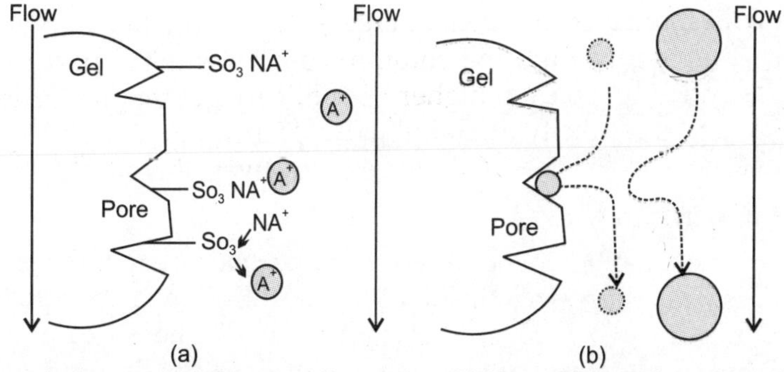

Schematic diagram depicting separation modes of (a) Ion exchange chromatography (amino acid A^+ changed with sodium ions Na^+) (b) Size exclusion chromatography.

Fig. 10.5: Separation mechanism of ion exchange and size exclusion chromatography

of refractive index detector is typical. This mode of chromatography is known as gel permeation or gel filtration chromatography too.

COMMON TERMS USED IN HPLC

Every system has its own parameters and special terms are used to describe these parameters. Of the separation modes, RPC is most widely used in pharmacy. Hence, terms associated with this process are described below.

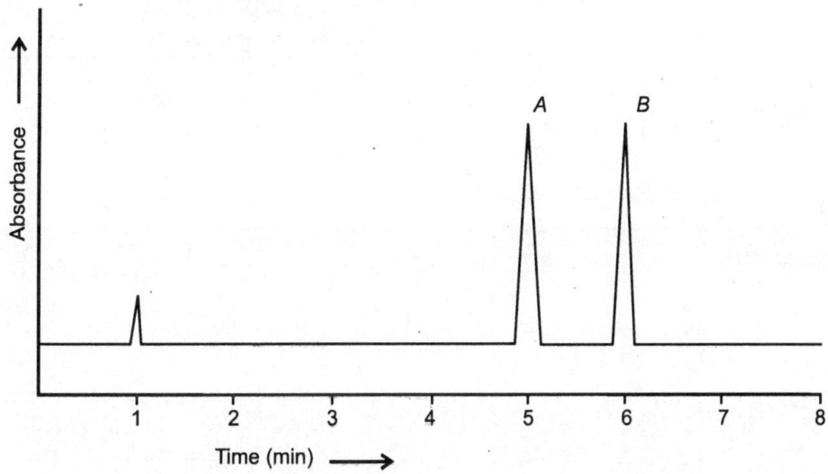

A chromatogram showing the retention time *A* and *B*

Fig. 10.6: Concept of retention time

Retention time (T_R): It is the most widely used term in RPC. Eluting molecules are identified on the basis of retention time, which is the time between sample injection and peak maxima. In Fig. 10.6, retention time recorded by the analytes *A* and *B* are 5 and 6 minutes respectively.

Void time (T_M): Void time is the residence time of a component, which is not retained by column. It is the time of first disturbance in the baseline caused by the sample solvent, which is also called hold up time. In Fig. 10.6, a small peak is observed at 1 minute. This peak indicates the hold up time is 1 minute.

Peak Height and Width (h, w_b)

The concentration of analytes is measured from the peak areas of the chromatograms. The height of the peak represents the highest concentration of the solute. Peak area is roughly equal to $1/2 \times w_b \times h$. The peak width is usually measured at the base (w_b) or peak half height. To measure the w_b, two tangent lines are drawn from the steepest inflection points of the peak. The distance between the two points at which the two tangents cut the baseline is w_b. The width at half height is easier to measure and is used for determination of column efficiency. The height or area of a peak is proportional to the amount of analyte. Since, it is difficult to measure peak width at the base, a relationship with width of half height is used (Fig. 10.7).

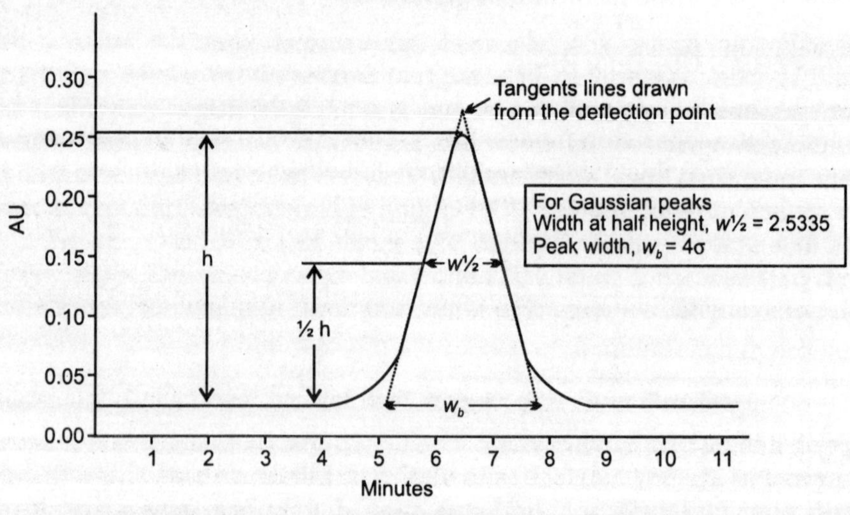

Fig. 10.7: Determination of height and width of a Gaussian peak

Peak volume: Popularly known as bandwidth, it is the volume of the mobile phase containing the peak. Peak volume is the volume of the mobile phase that passes through the detector when the peak is recorded. It is obtained by multiplying the flow rate (F) with peak width (w_b). For an eluting peak, greater the w_b, greater is the peak volume.

$$\text{Peak volume} = w_b \times F \qquad \text{(Eq. 10.1)}$$

So greater the height or lesser the peak volume or sharper will be the peak.

The Retention Volume (V_R)

It is the volume of mobile phase needed to elute an analyte at a given flow rate. The retention volume is found by multiplying the retention factor (T_R) with flow rate (F).

$$V_R = T_R \times F \qquad \text{(Eq. 10.2)}$$

Void volume **(V_M):** Void volume is the volume of the empty space within the column. It is the difference of total inside space of the column (internal volume) and the space occupied by packing. Hence, V_M is the sum of the inter-particle volume (V_0) and interstitial volume (V_e). V_e is the volume of the pores inside the solid support. For most of the columns, the void volume can be estimated by the equation:

$$V_M = 0.65\, V_c = 0.65\, \pi r^2 L \qquad \text{(Eq. 10.3)}$$

Where, V_c is the inner volume of the column, r is inner radius of the column and L represents the length of the column. Peak volume is proportional to V_M or void volume. As smaller columns have less void space, they produce less peak volumes.

Retention factor **(K):** Retention factor is expressed as the ratio of time, a solute resides in the stationary phase relative to the time it resides in the mobile phase. Retention factor is given by,

$$K = \frac{T_R - T_M}{T_M} \qquad \text{(Eq. 10.4)}$$

It is the degree of retention of the sample components in the column.

When a substance is not retained by the stationary phase it will elute at the same time as its solvent. The value of $(T_R - T_M)$ will be 0 and subsequently K will be 0. A value of $K > 20$ indicates that the sample is highly retained and process of elution may be impracticably long. A value of 1 to 20 is usually recommended for separation, as this gives the analytes sufficient time to interact with stationary phase and results in differential migration.

Peak Symmetry or Asymmetry Factor (A_s)

Ideally chromatographic peaks should be perfectly symmetrical. In reality, peaks can be slightly inclined at the front or end. The asymmetry factor is used to measure this tendency of deviation from symmetry. It is measured at the level of 10% peak height. In Fig. 10.8, the horizontal line drawn at 10% peak height has cut the peak at two points A and B. If the A and B represent the distance of this two points from the point of intersection, asymmetry factor A_s is defined by B/A.

Tailing Factor (T_f)

Peak tailing is a common defect caused by adsorption or extra column band broadening (adsorption of analytes other than the packing of column). Usually, polar interactions of the analytes with free silanol groups cause tailing by adsorbing some of the analytes and making them move more slowly to elute after the main band. On the other hand, if the quantity of the analytes loaded to the column is high, a fraction of analyte may elute early and fronting occurs. Tailing factor is very important for pharmaceutical analysis. If the value of T_f is 1.0, it indicates a perfectly symmetrical peak. $T_f > 2$ indicates a tailing peak, which is difficult to integrate for peak area and hence considered unacceptable.

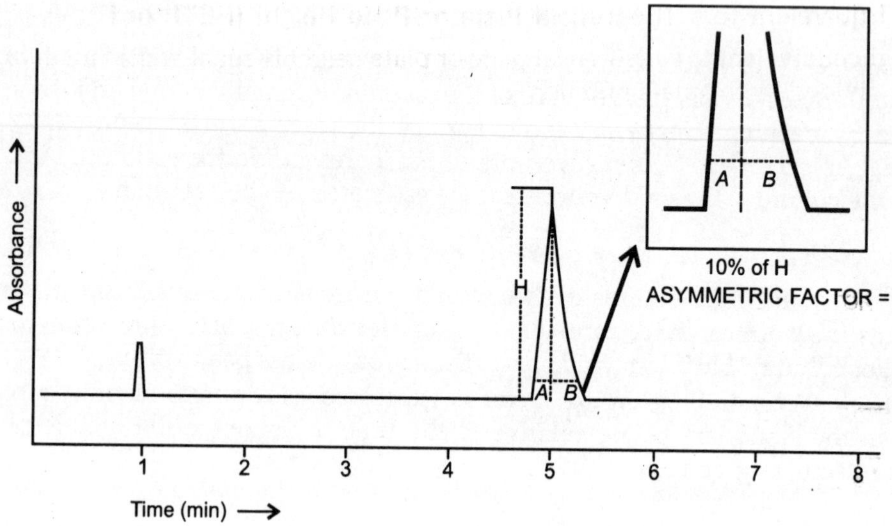

Fig. 10.8: Illustration of the asymmetry factors

Resolution (R_s)

One of the main functions of HPLC is separation of the components of a mixture and resolution is a measure of the degree of separation. Good resolution is obtained when retention time of the analytes is sufficiently different from one another and the peaks do not overlap in any way. Resolution time is defined as the difference of the retention time (of the two peaks) divided by the average peak width. If 2 analytes *A* and *B* in a mixture have retention times 6 and 7 minutes and have peak widths 0.15 and 0.25 minutes, the resolution will be the difference of the time (7–6 minute) divided by the average of the peak width [(0.15 + 0.25)/2]. Here the resolution factor is 5 (1.0/0.2 = 5). If $R_s = 0$, it indicates co-elution (coming out of the column together without any separation) when $R_s = 1$, peaks are perfectly separated.

Column Efficiency and Plate Number (N)

The concept of plate number and plate height has come from industrial distillation process. A long distillation column can accommodate many plates and concurrently can separate a mixture into many components. In HPLC, there are no discrete plates inside the columns but the concept of plate number and plate height can be used to indicate the efficiency of separation. An efficient column produces sharp peaks and can separate many samples in short time. The plate number (*N*) or the number of theoretical plates is a measure of the efficiency of the column. Plate number *N* is defined as the squared ratio of the retention time and the standard deviation of the peak. For a Guassian peak, i.e. a peak symmetrical in nature, w_b is equal to 4 standard deviation (σ) and number of the theoretical plates are calculated as,

$$N = (t_R/\sigma)^2 \qquad \text{(Eq. 10.5)}$$

Height Equivalent to a Theoretical Plate or Plate Height (HETP or H)

The height equivalent to a theoretical plate or plate height is equal to the length of the column divided by the plate number.

$$HETP = L/N \qquad \text{(Eq. 10.6)}$$

Where L is the length of the column and N, the plate number. The main controlling factor of plate height is the particle diameter (d_p). For a well-packed column, H is approximately equal to 2.5 d_p.

To clarify the concept let us take the example of two columns of same length—say 15 cm. Columns are packed with 10 and 5 micron particles respectively. So, the plate number of the first column is

$$\frac{15 \times 10000\,\mu}{2.5 \times 10\,\mu} = 6000.$$

But the second column will have plate number just the double of first column.

$$\frac{15 \times 10000\,\mu}{2.5 \times 5\,\mu} = 12000$$

Hence, the columns packed with smaller particles are more efficient in separating the mixtures.

HPLC SYSTEM

A typical HPLC system consists of a pump, an injector, a column, a detector and data interpretation device. However, modern HPLC systems also include column oven, online degasser and auto-samplers.

HPLC systems are basically of two types:

1. Modular, e.g. Aligent 1100 series, Jasco low pressure systems.
2. Integrated, e.g. Shimadzu, Waters.

Modular Systems

In modular systems, separately built standardized units are stacked together to form a system. This allows easy servicing. If a part gets damaged, replacement is easy.

Integrated Systems

In this type of systems, modules are built inside the single housings and are controlled by a single control board. Integrated systems usually have better overall performance as the modules work together with greater harmony but need more specialized maintenance.

Special systems: For research purpose HPLC has been merged with different identification devices and number special systems have come up.

LC NMR

LC NMR is a combination of HPLC and NMR. The traditional NMR needs pure sample for study and minimum sample requirement is in milligrams. Combination of HPLC and NMR allows identification of components from the mixture at low concentration levels. HPLC separates the mixture into single components, which are later identified by NMR. Similarly, HPLC can be coupled with infrared spectrophotometer and atomic absorption spectrometers to facilitate compound identification.

Preparative LC and Biopurification System

Synthetic chemists mainly use these types of systems. They use it for the separation of synthesized compounds, once the preparation is over. The quantity of sample is the main consideration in the choice of a preparative column. Preparative LC systems with bigger pumps deal with large flow rates and have wider internal channels. Eluents, which are rich in sample analytes, present a risk of signal saturation. Hence, detectors of such LC have short path lengths. Recent revolution in biotechnology has given birth to the branch of proteomics. Proteomics is defined as the study of full set of proteins encoded by a genome. Samples obtained from proteomics experiments are complex mixtures, which are difficult to be separated by HPLC alone. Hence, the concept of multi-dimensional chromatography has been developed. Here the samples are fractionated by first column and subsequently run into a second set of columns. The resolution is increased manifold by such techniques. Coupled with mass spectrophotometer and bioinformatics software, these 2-*D* systems can be powerful tools for the characterization of complex protein peptide mixtures. HPLC is used in High Throughput Screening (HTS) of drug discovery research too.

DIFFERENT PARTS OF HPLC SYSTEM

Figure 10.9 depicts different parts of HPLC system.

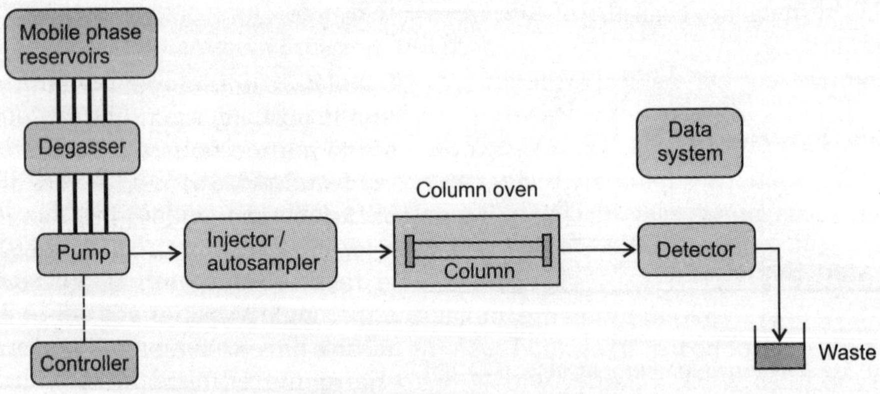

Fig. 10.9: Different parts of HPLC system

Pumps

Pump is one of the two most important parts of HPLC systems. It is the device that makes the mobile phase flow over the stationary phase. A typical solvent delivery system of HPLC uses reciprocating pump mechanism. Here a motorized cam drives a piston to deliver solvent through a set of check valves. A microprocessor coordinates the piston speed with other components. All components with which the solvent comes in contact are made of inert materials. For example, pump heads are made of stainless steel. Ruby balls and sapphire pistons are used in check valves, which come in intimate contact with the solvents to minimize the possibility of interaction. Specialized pumps are required for micro and nano systems. In systems used for biopurification and ion exchange chromatography, the fluidic components are produced from polyether-etherketone (PEEK) or titanium.

Use of modern binary high pressure mixing systems has increased the solvent selection capacity of HPLC. Each pump is connected to two-solvent reservoirs through an automated valve. Low-pressure mixing pumps are mainly used in research laboratories whereas high-pressure mixing pumps are used in LC/MS and HTS applications.

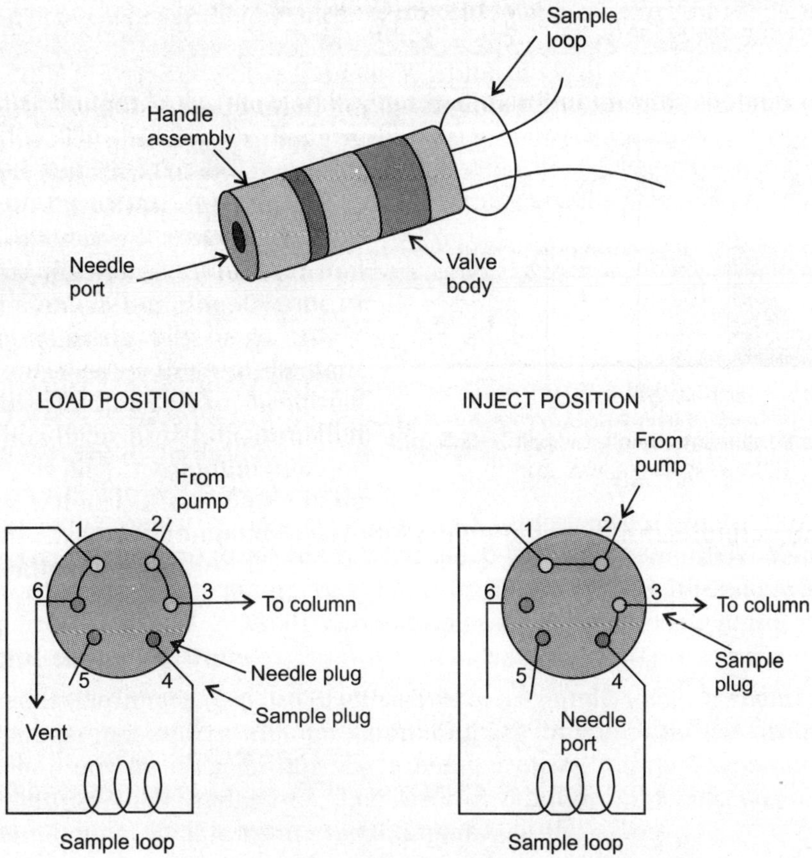

Fig. 10.10: Different parts of an injector

Injectors

Injectors introduce the sample into column under high pressure. A common injector is the Rheodyne model 7125 injector (Fig. 10.10). It consists of six-port valve with a rotor, a sample loop and an injector. Loop between port 1 and 4 connect it to pump which help in developing pressure, port 3 is attached to column, excess sample comes out from port 5 and 6. For manual injection, a 22 gauge blunt-tip needle is used to load a precise quantity of sample into the sample loop at the 'Load' position. The sample is delivered to the column by switching the valve into inject position.

Auto samplers reduce the cost of operation because sampling is done automatically from sample vials through a motorized injection valve and moving sampling needles. The moving syringe can draw samples or flush solvents depending on the position of solenoid valves. A microprocessor synchronizes the movement of syringe and timings of injection sequence. In another design, sample vials are brought to the sampling needle by a set of robotic arms.

Column

The HPLC column is the heart of HPLC system. A wide variety of HPLC columns have been developed to cater to the needs of different types of separation. However, in pharmacy, reverse phase columns are mainly used.

A typical HPLC column is a thin tube usually made of stainless steel. The tube is filled with small particles that retard the movement of analytes and split the sample into a series of distinct bands because of its varying affinity for the different components of sample. Columns can be classified according to their size, separation modes and support types.

The columns used in pharmacy for analytical work are usually of reverse phase separation mode. Dimensionwise they are 50 to 250 mm long, 2.0 to 4.6 mm in internal diameter, packed with small (3, 5 or 10 μm) C_{18} silica-based bonded phase. Operating pressure ranges from 500 to 3000 psi. Irrespective of separation modes, columns need to be replaced periodically. Typical column life is 500–2000 injections.

Figure 10.11 shows the end-fitting has a narrow opening through which the column is connected to a thinner tube. The usual outer diameter of the column is 4.6 mm and the narrow connecting tubes are of 1.6 mm (outer diameter). Through these narrow tubes the column is connected to the injector where the sample is fed. The fine particles inside the columns are tightly packed and held in place with a set of microporous end

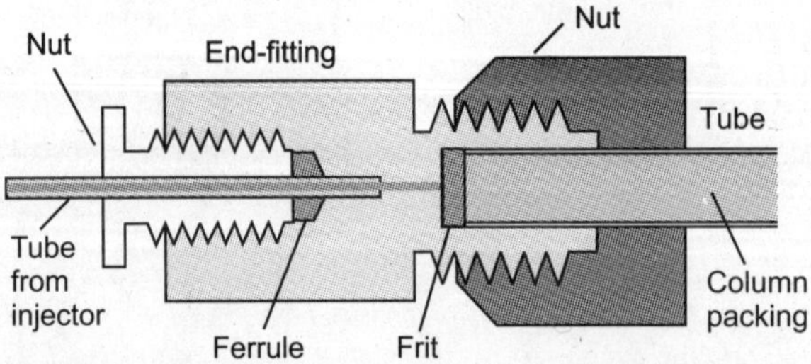

Schematic of the inlet of a standard HPLC column showing details on the inlet tube with compression screw and ferrule, the end-fitting, and the inlet frit.

Fig. 10.11: Different parts of a typical HPLC column

frits. The pore diameter of the microporous frits (2 μm) is lesser than the size of the packing materials so that the packing cannot slip through the pores.

Sample and mobile phase, while flowing through the column, come in intimate contact with its inner surface. As these materials have high solvent property, to minimize the risk of corrosion, column body is made of high quality stainless steel. For highly reactive samples as in ion chromatography greater precaution is taken. Instead of stainless steel, column bodies are made of polyetheretherketone (PEEK) or titanium, which are highly corrosion resistant.

Sometimes, columns come in cartridges. The systems contain permanent holders and like the refill cartridges of ballpoint pens, cartridge columns are fixed within the holder with the help of pressed-in frits.

Column packings are usually silica-based. Surface silanol group in the silica is the major problem in the analysis of basic analytes. Silica materials usually have metallic contamination and such silica is extremely acidic. To prevent adsorption of basic analytes, usually amines (triethyl amine) are used in the mobile phase. High purity silica with less than 50 ppm of metals can improve the separation dramatically. Use of hybrid particles can also reduce tailing. These materials can withstand wide pH range.

Polar-Embedded Groups

Polar groups, e.g. carbamate, urea, amide, ether, sulphonamide, inserted into the hydrophobic chains can shield silanols. The columns made with such packings are less retentive of neutral and basic analytes compared to their C_{18} or C_8 counterparts. Highly polar moieties are retained by polar-embedded phases. Partially bonded high-purity silica support can also be used for highly polar substances, e.g. Alltech platinum EPS and Water Atlantis dC_{18}. Table 10.1 gives characteristics of some modern HPLC columns.

Table 10.1: Characteristics of some modern HPLC columns

Manufacturer	*Packing (stationary phase)*	*Surface area* (m^2/g)	*Pore size*
Aligent	Zorbax	300	70
Bischoff	ProntoSil	100	300
Eka Chemicals	Kromasil	340	100
Machery Nagel	Nucleosil 100	350	100
Merck KGaA	Chromolith	300	130
Merck KGaA	LiChrospher	350	100
Phenomenex	Gemini	375	110*
Varian	Polaris	180	180

Information taken from reference of Michaeal W. Dong.
* Hybrid column.
Note that for small pore size packing, surface area is high.

Guard Columns

As the name indicates, guard columns actually protect or guard the main column from contamination and increase its lifetime. Basically, a guard column is a small column placed before an analytical column. In pharmaceutical experiments, often samples of biological origin, e.g. blood, tissue extracts, etc. are analyzed. These samples are usually small in volume and difficult to clean up. If they are fed into the main column directly, they may contaminate the packing materials and may be retained into the column. Use of guard column is recommended for such dirty samples. Usually, guard columns are packed with the same materials as the main analytical column. Attaching guard column helps in sample cleaning but they should not cause significant increase in operating pressure. Sometimes, a special type of guard column known as 'scavenger column' is placed between the pump and injector. Here rather than cleaning of sample, the purpose is to protect the analytical column from mobile phase contaminants. Columns that use extremely small particles as packing material get clogged easily. While passing through the scavenger column, mobile phases get cleaned up and chance of clogging is reduced.

Detectors

While the column separates the complex mixture into simple solutions, the detector measures the concentrations of these solutions (eluting analytes). The detector recognizes the analytes by monitoring one of its inherent properties. UV/Vis and photodiode array detectors are among the most commonly used detectors.

UV/Vis detectors: UV/Visual detectors measure the absorption of UV or visible light by HPLC eluents. As most of pharmaceuticals show UV absorption, this detector is widely used in Pharmacy. It usually consists of a deuterium lamp (radiation source), a monochromator (movable gratings or prism that allows only lights of particular wavelength to pass through the exit slit) and a small flow cell through which the mobile phase flows. Normally, dual beam design is used. The light generated by the lamp is divided into two halves, of which only one half flows through the sample cell. Intensity of the both the beams is measured by separate photodiodes. In contrast to normal spectrophotometers, which have bigger flow cells (1–3 ml), flow cells used in HPLC units are small in volume. Typical volume of HPLC flow cells at 2–10 μL and path length is 2–10 μm. Usually, high quality quartz cells are used.

Quantification is done by measuring the absorbance, which is defined as the negative logarithm of transmittance. It is the ratio of the transmitted light to that of incident light. When 90% light is absorbed, absorbance value is 1. The benchmark noise level is typically $1.0 \pm \times 10^{-5}$. The high end of linear absorption range is typically set at 1 to 1.5 but modern and sophisticated instruments have lower noise level and extended high ends (maximum absorbance measurable). The sensitivity of measurement depends on extinction coefficients of the analytes. Higher the extinction, greater is the sensitivity of the method (Table 10.2).

Photodiode Array Detectors (PDA)

In contrast to single wavelength detectors, which record the absorption at single wavelength, PDA detectors provide complete UV spectra of eluting peaks. In short, it performs as a multi-wavelength UV/Vis absorbance detector and is preferred for method development. In UV/Vis detector, the spectrum of deuterium lamp is grated

Table 10.2: Light absorption properties of some important chromophoric groups

Chromophore	λ_{max} *(nm)*	*Extinction coefficient* (ε)
Carbonyl	280	16
Alkyne	225	160
Amido	214	41
Azo	339	5
Nitro	280	22
Carboxyl	204	41
Nitrate	270	12
Conjugated olefins	217–250	> 20,000
Ketone	282	27
Alkylated benzenes	250–260	200–300
Phenol	270	1,450
Aniline	280	1,430
Napthalene	286	9,300
Styrene	244	12,000

* Data extracted from reference of Michaeal W. Dong

into single wavelength and light of a particular wavelength passes through the flow cell. In PDA detector (Fig. 10.12), the entire spectrum of the deuterium lamp passes through the flow cell onto a diode array element that measures the intensity of light at each wavelength. Most PDAs use charge-coupled diode array. Spectral evaluation software can determine concentration of chromatographic entities (separated into different bands) as well as spectrum* of each entity separated. In short, the modern PDA detectors can show 3-*D* spectral display of overall evaluation of entire sample.

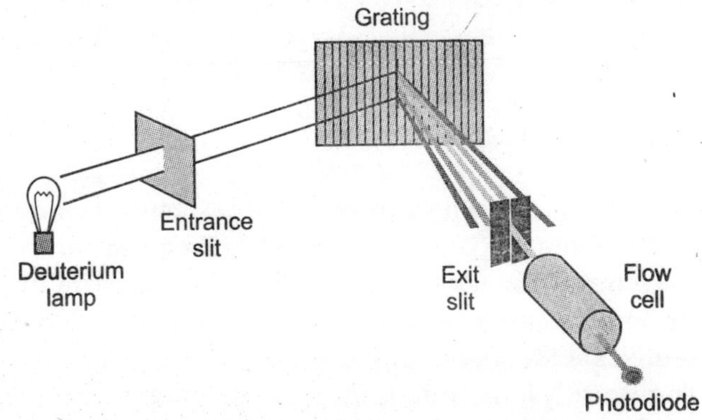

A diagram of UV-visible absorbance photodiode detector

Fig. 10.12: Photodiode detector

Fluorescence detector (Fig. 10.13) is useful only for eluents, which show the property of fluorescence. The fluorescence detector measures the intensity of the emitted florescent light of the eluents at right angle to that of the excitatory light. It is extremely sensitive and low concentrations like picogram or femtogram (10^{-12}, 10^{-15} g) can be measured.

A fluorescence detector has all the components of a regular fluorimeter—a xenon emission source to generate radiation, an excitation monochromator that selects the excitatory radiation, a square flow cell that directs the emitted radiation at right angle to excitatory radiation, emission monochromator and a photo multiplier that amplifies the emitted photons. In low-cost units, filters are used instead of monochromators.

More expensive units have double monochromators that are capable of detecting multiple components.

Refractive Index Detectors (RID)

Refractive index detectors (Fig. 10.14) measure the difference in refractive index between pure solvents and eluting analyte. However, these are not useful in gradient elution. The reference cell is flushed with pure solvent and sample cell contains solution

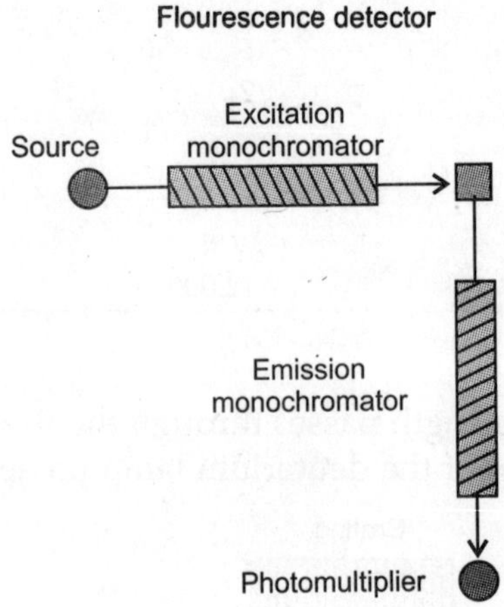

Fig. 10.13: Fluorescence detector

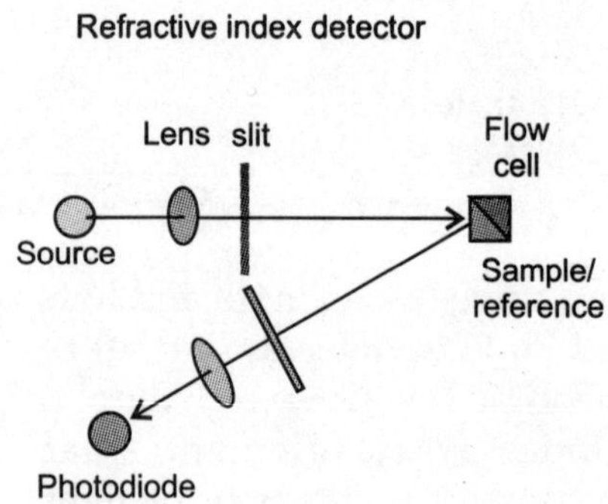

Fig. 10.14: Refractive index detector

of analyte. Since a solution is sure to have a different refractive index from that of a pure solvent, RID detectors are universal in nature. The main disadvantage with this detector lies in its low sensitivity (can measure up to the concentration of 0.01 to 0.1 µg/ml). It cannot measure the difference of refractive index if the concentration of eluted substance is low. Analytes, which have low chromophoric activities like sugar, triglycerides, organic acids, polymers, etc. are measured by these detectors. As the devices of this type are prone to temperature and flow changes, flow cells are thermostated for improving the sensitivity of detection.

Chemiluminescence Nitrogen Detector (CLND)

CLND is a special detector, which can be used for detecting nitrogen substances. In this, nitrogen-containing substances are oxidized to nitric oxide by the pyro-chemiluminescence technology. Nitric oxide generated in the reaction then reacts with ozone to yield a specific light. The quantity of light emitted is directly proportional to the quantity of nitrogen present. This detector does not allow the use of nitrogen containing mobile phase like acetonitrile.

Electrochemical Detector (ECD)

The basic principle in this type of detection is the measurement of an electric current generated by an analyte. The eluent coming from the column passes through a flow cell, which contains electrodes. Electro-active analytes generate electric current. Sensitive detection is possible up to the picogram level. Catecholamines, reducing sugars, compounds containing OH, NH_2, diazo and nitro functional groups can be detected by this method. Commonly used electrodes are carbon, silver, gold, platinum, etc. Fouling of electrodes can be a real problem for this type of detectors.

Conductivity Detectors (CD)

It is mainly used in ion chromatography. It measures the electrical conductivity of the eluent stream, which contains ions, organic acids or surfactants.

Radiometric Detectors (RD)

This detector can be used when the HPLC eluents contain radioactive molecules. Usually, the phosphors caused by radionuclides are detected by liquid scintillation technology. This detector is used in experiments with tritium or C-14 labeled samples obtained from pharmacokinetic and toxicological analysis.

FACTORS AFFECTING SEPARATION

HPLC can simultaneously separate and estimate concentrations of individual components of a mixture. The efficacy of this separation is indicated by separation factor. If a sample has two components *A* and *B* and retention factors of these are K_a and K_b, the separation factor (α) is K_a/K_b. Selectivity must be greater than 1 for peak separation. Selectivity is dependent on many factors like nature of stationary phase, the composition of the mobile phase and properties of the analytes. A method developer studies all these factors and designs the method that shows optimum separation.

Mobile Phase

Mobile phase is the main weapon in the hand of a method developer to cause effective separation. Choice of mobile phase depends on the nature of the analytes. Mobile phase carries the analytes through the column and hence, analytes must be soluble in the mobile phase. Composition of the mobile phase is varied to change the selectivity.

As most of the HPLC systems use UV detector, it is desired that mobile phases should be UV transparent (not absorb UV light). They should also be non-corrosive, so that no interaction takes place with the column material. Other requirements are non-toxicity, non-inflammability, high purity and low cost. Commonly used solvents in HPLC system are methanol, acetonitrile (ACN), methylene chloride, water and *n*-hexane. Preparation of the mobile phase needs special care. When water is mixed with ethanol, the total volume is less than the sum total of 2 solvent volumes. So, in isocratic analysis, components of the mobile phase should be measured separately and then mixed. Mobile phase should be filtered before running into the column and usually 0.45 µm membrane filters are used. For filtration of aqueous solvents, cellulose acetate filter is used whereas nylon filter is used for organic solvents.

Special Components of Mobile Phase

Sometimes, natural affinity of an analyte for the stationary phase is not sufficient for effective binding and analytes are eluted before effective separation can take place. Hence, in such cases effective separation can be obtained by adding special molecules in the mobile phase. Long chain alkyl sulphonates can combine with basic analytes. Under acidic pH condition, basic analytes are ionized. Hence, for such analytes if the mobile phase contains sulphonate groups, ionized basic moieties will react with acidic sulphonates to form neutral ion pair. Such ion pairs because of their neutrality will be having higher affinity for the hydrophobic stationary phase of RPLC and retention of the analytes would be proportional to the length of the hydrophobic chain of the ion-pairing agent and its concentration. Tetraalkyl ammonium salts are used as ion-pairing agent for acidic analytes whereas alkyl sulphonates are used for basic analytes. Basic analytes are unionized at higher pH and better retained by stationary phases at higher pH. However, silica support has a limitation of pH. It dissolves when the pH is below 2 or above 8. Hence, hybrid particles, which are stable at higher pH, are used for such separation.

Solvent Strength and Selectivity

Solvent strength is related to polarity and selectivity also depends on the mode of chromatography used. Nonpolar hexane is a weak solvent in NPC whereas water is a strong solvent. The opposite is true for RPLC where the stationary phase is hydrophobic. Here water is a weak solvent and hexane is a strong solvent. Since, the stationary phase is hydrophobic in RPLC, it binds the lipophilic moieties and lipophilic hexane is able to remove it from the stationary phase much faster than water. Hence, water is a weak solvent for organic compounds. In RPLC solvent strength decreases in the following order; THF > ACN > EtOH > water (Table 10.3).

Table 10.3: Properties of some commonly used HPLC solvents

Solvent	*Solvent strength (E°)*	*Boiling point °C*	*Viscosity (cP) at 20° C*	*UV transparency upto (nm)*	*Refractive index*
n-Hexane	0.01	69	0.31	190	1.37
Toluene	0.29	78	0.59	285	1.49
Methylene chloride	0.42	40	0.44	233	1.42
Tetrahydrofuran	0.45	66	0.55	212	1.41
Acetonitrile	0.55–0.65	82	0.37	190	1.34
2-propanol	0.82	82	2.30	205	1.38
Methanol	0.95	65	0.54	205	1.33
Water	Very high	100	1.00	< 190	1.33

* Data extracted from reference of Michaeal W. Dong.

For example, reverse phase chromatography is used for the separation of two lipophilic moieties *A* and *B*. If ACN is used as the mobile phase they elute together because both are soluble in it. But when a mixture of 30% ACN and 70% water is used, the polarity of the mobile phase changes and the peaks are well separated. At 20% ACN the peaks are even more distant and clear-cut separation is observed. As a rule, molecules with lower lipophilicity elute faster. In general, increase in the strength of mobile phase by addition of organic solvent, decreases retention time in RPLC. A useful rule of thumb is that a 10% decrease in the organic solvent in the mobile phase produces a three fold increase in the retention time.

Buffers

Most of the drugs are weakly acidic or basic in nature. Extent of ionization for such molecules depends on the pH of the environment. Hence, if pH were such that a fraction of the analyte is ionized, it would be having lesser binding to the hydrophobic phase compared to the unionized fraction. Since the retention time depends on the extent of binding, the ionized fraction will elute faster than the unionized fraction. So for the same moiety, there is a chance of getting two peaks or at least a mixed peak. To prevent this, mobile phase is adjusted to a pH, which normally suppresses the ionization. Buffers are used to control the pH of the mobile phase. Selection of the buffers is done on the basis of their pKa, as buffering capacity is maximum within ± 1.5 pH units of pKa. However, the buffers should be used sparingly, as they absorb UV light to some extent (UV detector is widely used in HPLC systems). The recommended concentration of the buffer is 10 to 20 mM though higher concentration up to 50 mM is also used. For Mass spectrophotometers, volatile buffers are required. Buffers of ammonium salts are volatile in nature and are usually used for this purpose. Acidic mobile phases are mostly suitable for the determination of weakly acidic substances because they suppress ionization of analytes and they are strongly retained by the hydrophobic stationary phases of RPLC. Commonly used acids are phosphoric acid, trifluoroacetic acid and formic acid. Low pH mobile phases also suppress ionization of the surface silanol groups of silica support. This minimizes the tailing of peaks.

Flow Rate

Operating flow rate usually depends on column diameter. It is proportional to the square of the column's inner diameter. Smaller columns have lesser flow rate. Increasing the flow rate decreases the retention time but decreases the column performance. In isocratic analysis, composition of the mobile phase is kept constant. Here, the flow rate has no impact on retention factor or selection of column. Higher column temperature lowers viscosity of the mobile phase. This decreases column's backpressure. As the solubility of the mobile phase is affected at higher temperature, retention efficiency and selectivity are also affected.

The degree of separation (R_s) between two solutes is given by the following equation:

$$R_s = \left(\frac{K}{K+1}\right)\left(\frac{\alpha - 1}{\alpha}\right)\frac{\sqrt{N}}{4} \qquad \text{(Eq. 10.6)}$$

As K value increases, $K/K+1$ approaches 1. Hence, higher K value is beneficial. However, for K values greater than 10, the difference becomes insignificant.

Selectivity depends on stationary and mobile phase character. Selectivity is proportional to $(\alpha - 1)/\alpha$. Hence, mobile phase adjustment is a powerful tool in maximizing the resolution. Similarly, use of a longer column as well as smaller particle size can be helpful.

Band Broadening

The Van Deemter equation was developed to explain the phenomenon of band broadening. It shows the relationship of linear flow with plate height. As velocity decreases plate height increases. At lower velocity, plate height is more and enough time is allowed for proper partitioning. But at very low flow velocity, separation time may be impractically long. Again at higher flow rate, the plate height increases. The lowest inflection in the curve shows the optimum flow rate and minimum particle size.

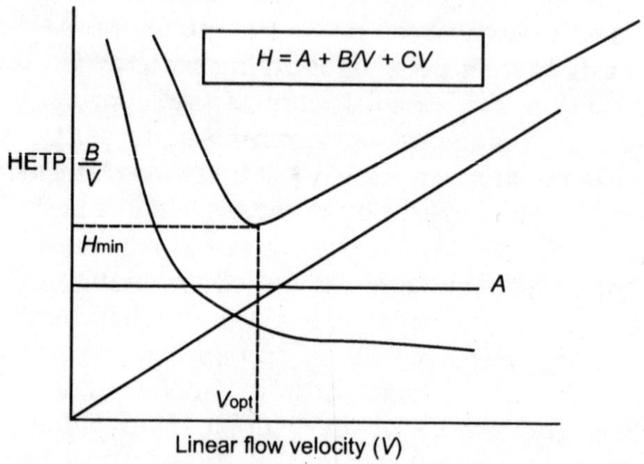

Van Deemter curve showing the relationship of HETP Vs average linear film velocity. H_{min} = linear plate height, V_{opt} = optimum velocity.

Fig. 10.15: Relationship of flow velocity with plate height

$$H = A + \frac{B}{V} + CV \qquad \text{(Eq. 10.7)}$$

The topmost curve of Fig. 10.15 is a composite curve, formed by the contribution of the three terms A, B/V and CV. The lower three curves marked with A, CV and B/V show the individual contribution of these factors.

A = Represents Eddy's diffusion term or multiple path diffusion. While passing through the column, instead of going forward, a fraction of the analytes may travel backwards or sidewards. Low flow rate or bigger particle packing leads to high A values.

B = Longitudinal diffusion of the solute band in the mobile phase and is proportional to the diffusivity of the solute.

C = Resistance to mass transfer due to time lags and due to slow diffusion of the mobile phase into stationary phase. It is proportional to dp^2/D_m. As dp^2 is much lesser in columns packed with fine particles, finer particles give better separation.

V = Linear flow velocity.

Isocratic analysis is done for separation of sample mixtures whereas in gradient analysis strength of the mobile phase is increased with time. Gradient analysis is preferred for analysis of complex mixtures.

SAFETY FACTORS OF HPLC

For analytical purposes, mobile phases used in HPLC are of small volume. As the flow rates are moderate, safety hazards due to the inflammable material is low. However, high electric voltage is required for operation of the machine. A large mobile phase bottle, kept close to a machine, involves the risk of explosion if inflammable. Some mobile phases like tetrahydrofuran, methylene chloride, DMSO, DMF should be used with proper caution. Volatile and toxic substances should be handled under a laboratory fume hood. During vacuum filtration there is a potential danger of flask implosion. Vacuum grade glassware should be used to minimize this risk.

BIBLIOGRAPHY

1. Alfonso R Gennaro (Chief Editor), *Remington Science and Practice of Pharmacy*, 20th ed., published by Philadelphia College of Pharmacy, Philadelphia, 2000.
2. DG Watson, *Pharmaceutical Analysis*, 2nd ed., Elsevier Limited, 2005.
3. KA Connor's, *A Textbook of Pharmaceutical Analysis*, Wiley Interscience Publishers, New York, 1999.
4. Michael W. Dong, Modern HPLC for Practising Scientists, Wiley Interscience Publishers, 2006.
5. Willard et. al., *Instrumental Method of Analysis*, CBS Publishers & Distributors, 6th ed., Delhi, 1996.

11 Nuclear Magnetic Resonance Spectroscopy

THEORY OF NUCLEAR MAGNETIC RESONANCE

Nuclear magnetic resonance spectroscopy is the analytical method to find out the number of magnetically distinct atoms in a given compound. All the atoms contain nuclei and all the nuclei contain charge. Some of the charged nuclei possess 'spin'. They are those nuclei which contain either an odd atomic number or odd atomic mass or both, e.g. ${}^{1}_{1}H$, ${}^{2}_{1}H$, ${}^{13}_{6}C$, ${}^{14}_{7}N$, ${}^{17}_{8}O$,${}^{35}_{17}Cl$, etc. The nuclei which have even number of atomic mass and charge are not suitable for NMR spectroscopy, e.g. ${}^{12}_{6}C$, ${}^{16}_{8}O$, etc. Those nuclei which possess spin, they spin on their nuclear axis which generates a magnetic dipole 'μ'. The angular momentum of this spinning charge can be quantified and described in terms of quantum spin number 'I'. Angular momemtum of a particle about an origin is a vector quantity (i.e. a directional quantity) related to rotation or spin, and is equal to the mass of the particle multiplied by the cross product of the position vector of the particle with its velocity vector. The angular momentum of a system of particles is the sum of that of the particles within it. For each nucleus there are $2I + 1$ allowed spin states with integral differences ranging from $-I$ to $+ I$, i.e. $+I$, $(I - 1) - (-I + 1)$, $-I$.

For example, $I = \frac{1}{2}$ for hydrogen and allowed spin states are $+\frac{1}{2}$ and $-\frac{1}{2}$.

For chlorine atom $I = \frac{3}{2}$, therefore, allowed spin states are $+\frac{3}{2}, +\frac{1}{2}, -\frac{1}{2}, -\frac{3}{2}$.

These spin states have equal amount of energy (degenerated) in the absence of a magnetic field. But when a magnetic field is applied these protons possessing spin and there own magnetic field align themselves either with or opposite to the applied magnetic field. For example, ${}^{1}_{1}H$ atom has $+\frac{1}{2}$ and $-\frac{1}{2}$ spin state. The protons which have spin state of $+\frac{1}{2}$ align themselves with the field (hence comparatively lower energy), and those who have $-\frac{1}{2}$ spin state align themselves opposite to the field (therefore, comparatively higher energy), Figs 11.1 and 11.2. Hence, the external magnetic field has split the spin state into higher and lower level (Fig. 11.3).

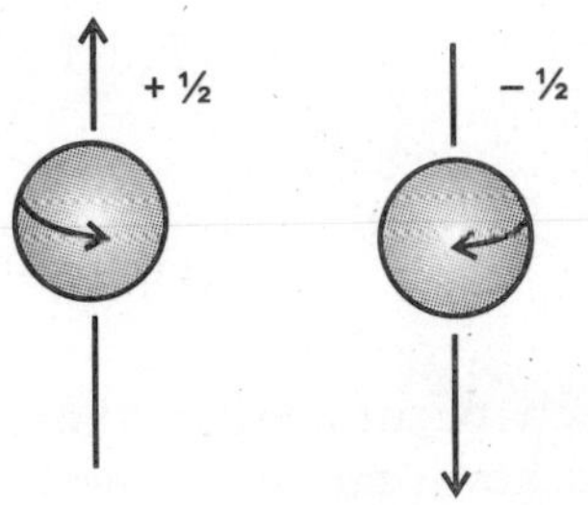

Fig. 11.1: Two spin states allowed for proton

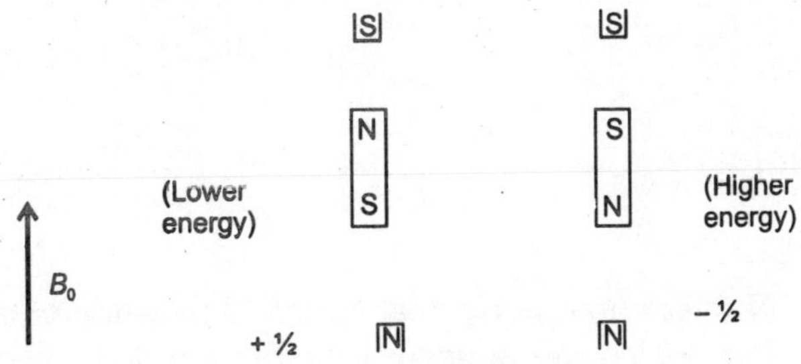

Fig. 11.2: Two arrangements of bar magnets—aligned (lower energy) and opposed (higher energy)

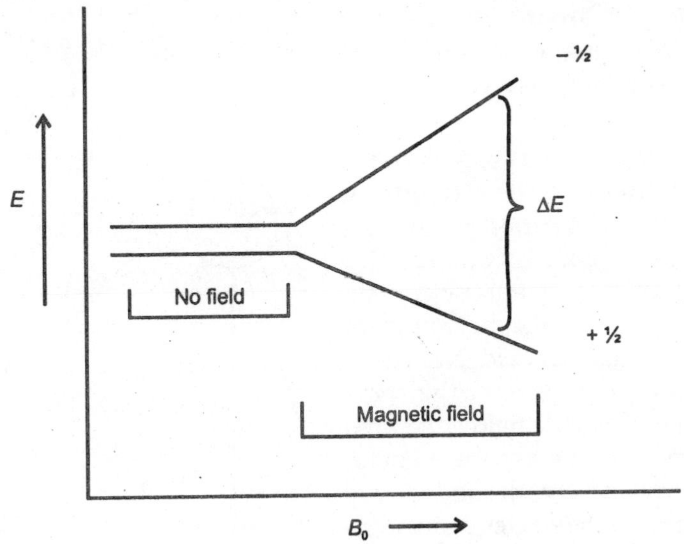

Fig. 11.3: Change in the spin-state energy separation with increase in applied magnetic field, B_0.

Stronger the applied magnetic field, greater will be the difference between the spin states,

$$\Delta E = f(B_0) \tag{Eq. 11.1}$$

as $E_{absorbed}(\Delta E)$ = difference in the energy levels of two opposite energy states = $h\nu$.

Each nucleus depending on its charge and mass has its own magnetogyric ratio 'γ' which is the ratio of magnetic dipole moment to angular momentum, and it is constant for each nucleus, therefore,

$$\Delta E = f(\gamma B_0) = h\nu \tag{Eq. 11.2}$$

As the angular momentum has units of $h/2\pi$, the above equation becomes

$$\Delta E = \gamma \left(\frac{h}{2\pi}\right) B_0 = h\nu \qquad \text{(Eq. 11.3)}$$

$$\nu = \left(\frac{\gamma}{2\pi}\right) B_0 \qquad \text{(Eq. 11.4)}$$

Nuclear magnetic resonance is a phenomenon which occurs when those nuclei which are aligned with the applied magnetic field are induced to absorb energy and change their spin state to opposite one, this is known as resonance. To understand this phenomenon we have to consider the spinning nuclei as a top which when spinned under the influence of applied magnetic field possess two motions; one is spin around its axis, and second one is wobbling as shown in Figs 11.4 (a) and 11.4 (b) respectively.

This wobbling for a proton is termed as *precessing*. The frequency of precession is directly proportional to the strength of applied magnetic field. Since proton is a charged particle its precession (angular frequency, ω) generates an oscillating electric field around it of the same frequency as that of applied magnetic field. Now if we supply a radiowave of exactly the same frequency as that of electric field generated by precessing proton, the two frequencies (radio and electric) can couple, and energy can be transferred to the nucleus causing a change in spin which is termed as resonance (Fig. 11.5).

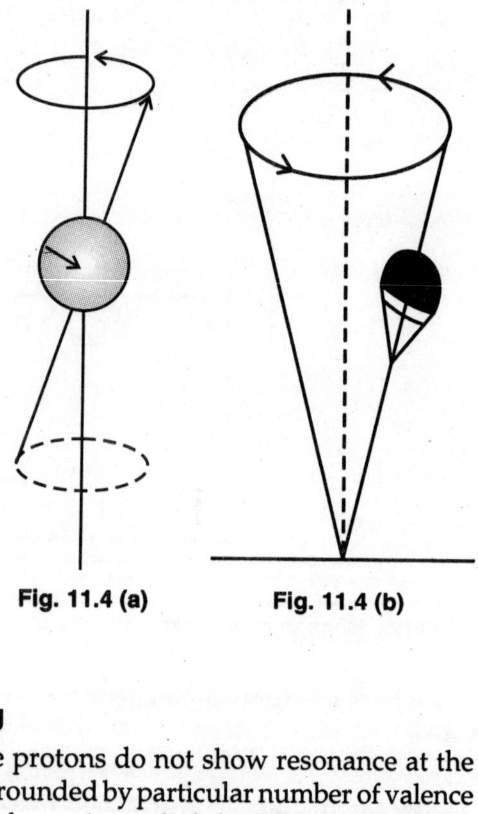

Fig. 11.4 (a) **Fig. 11.4 (b)**

Chemical Shift, Shielding and Deshielding

The utility of NMR lies in the fact that all the protons do not show resonance at the same frequency. It is so because protons are surrounded by particular number of valence electrons which vary from atom to atom, thus they exist in slightly different electronic environment from one another. When a magnetic field is applied the electrons present in the valence shell start circulating, this circulation known as local diamagnetic current, generates a counter magnetic field which opposes the applied magnetic field (Fig. 11.6). This effect is known as *diamagnetic shielding* or *diamagnetic anisotropy*. The diamagnetic shielding reduces the total strength of applied magnetic field which is reaching to the electron-embedded proton. More the number of valence electrons, more is the shielding and, therefore, lower is the strength of magnetic field being experienced by the proton. Lesser the strength of magnetic field experienced by the proton, lesser will be the precessing frequency, and hence, it will show resonance at lower frequency.

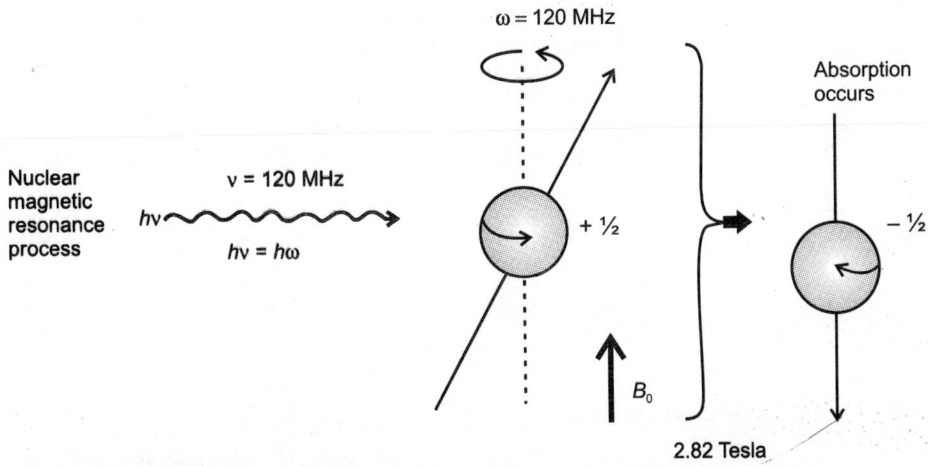

Fig. 11.5: The process of resonance in NMR; absorption occurs when ν = ω

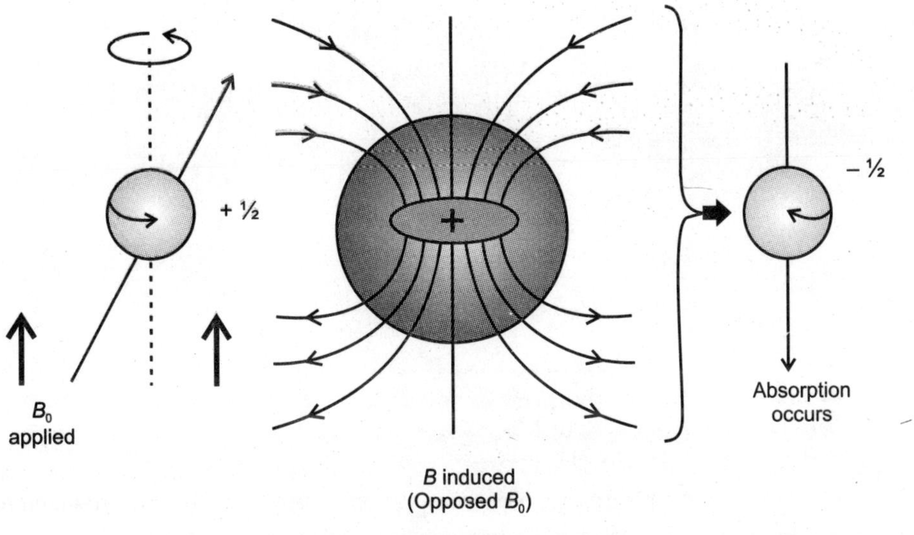

Fig. 11.6: Diamagnetic anisotropy

Thus, precessing frequency of a proton depends on the number of electrons in the valence shell also. Each proton in a molecule is in a slightly different chemical environment and consequently has a slightly different amount of electric shielding which results in a slightly different resonance frequency.

In NMR spectroscopy tetramethyl silane, $(CH_3)_4Si$, or TMS is used as standard reference as all the protons of methyl group are uniformly and more shielded than those of the most other known compounds. The resonance of the protons in the compound to be analyzed are reported in terms of how far they have shifted from those of TMS. As the NMR spectrometers are of variable range, e.g. 60 MHz, 120 MHz, 300 MHz, etc. there can be variation in the spectrum of the same compound obtained from different instruments. To overcome this discrepancy the signals are reported in field-independent measure called chemical shift (δ), which is

$$\delta = \frac{\text{Shift in Hz}}{\text{Spectrometer frequency in MHz}} \qquad \text{(Eq. 11.5)}$$

INSTRUMENTATION

1. Continuous Wave (CW) Instrument

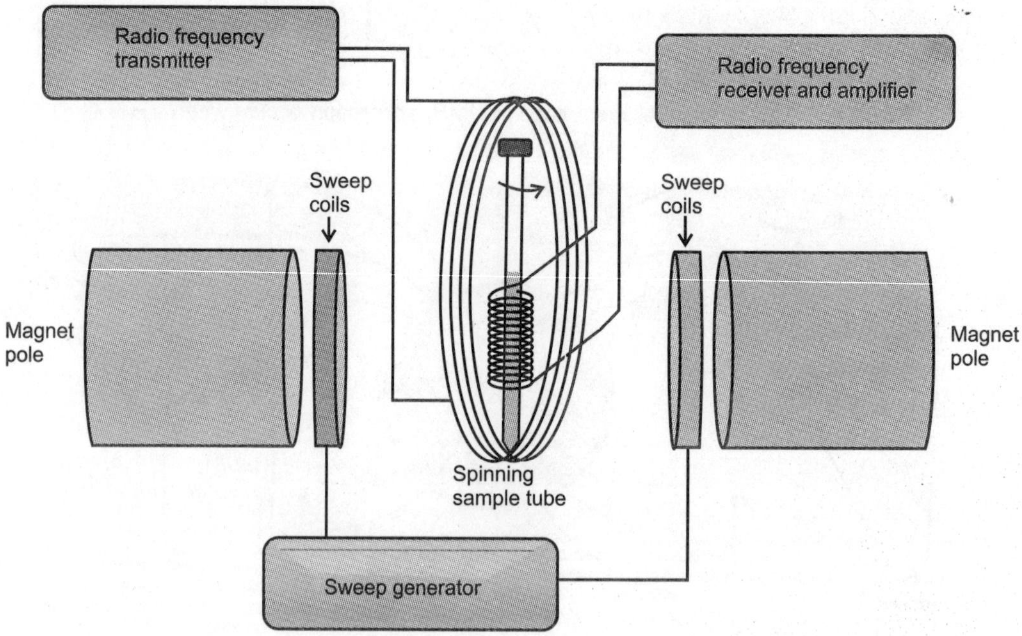

Fig. 11.7: A layout of the elements present in nuclear magnetic resonance spectrometer

The sample to be analyzed is put in a long cylindrical glass tube especially made for NMR. The sample is first dissolved in a proton-free solvent like $CDCl_3$ or CCl_4 and then a small amount of TMS is added as internal reference. The sample tube is placed in the gap between the two magnetic poles. In this gap where the sample tube is placed, a coil is attached there to a specific radiofrequency (e.g. 60 MHz) generator. This coil will supply the electromagnetic energy required to change the spin orientation of the proton. The detector coil is placed perpendicular to the RF oscillator coil. This coil detects the radiofrequency signal when resonance occurs. In an NMR instrument there are two energy variation sources—one is RF oscillator and the other one is magnetic field strength. In a typical NMR spectrophotometer generally the RF signal is kept constant and magnetic field strength is varied, e.g. in 60 MHz NMR instrument.

As the magnetic field strength is increased, the precessional frequencies of all protons increase. When the precessional frequency of a given type of proton reaches 60 MHz, it undergoes resonance.

As the strength of magnetic field is increased linearly (say, from 1.41 Tesla it can be increased upto 20 ppm) the recorder pen travels across the chart. From left to right (Fig. 11.10) the magnetic filed is increasing thus the protons which achieve resonance faster, i.e. those are deshielded appear on the left side (downfield), whereas those which are shielded more they appear on the right side (upfield) of the chart in the form of peaks. TMS is shown at a peak value of $\delta = 0$ ppm.

These types of instruments in which magnetic field is slowly increased, i.e. they scan from downfield to upfield end are known as continuous wave (CW) instruments (Fig. 11.7). Figure 11.8 shows an actual photograph of 800 MHz NMR spectrometer.

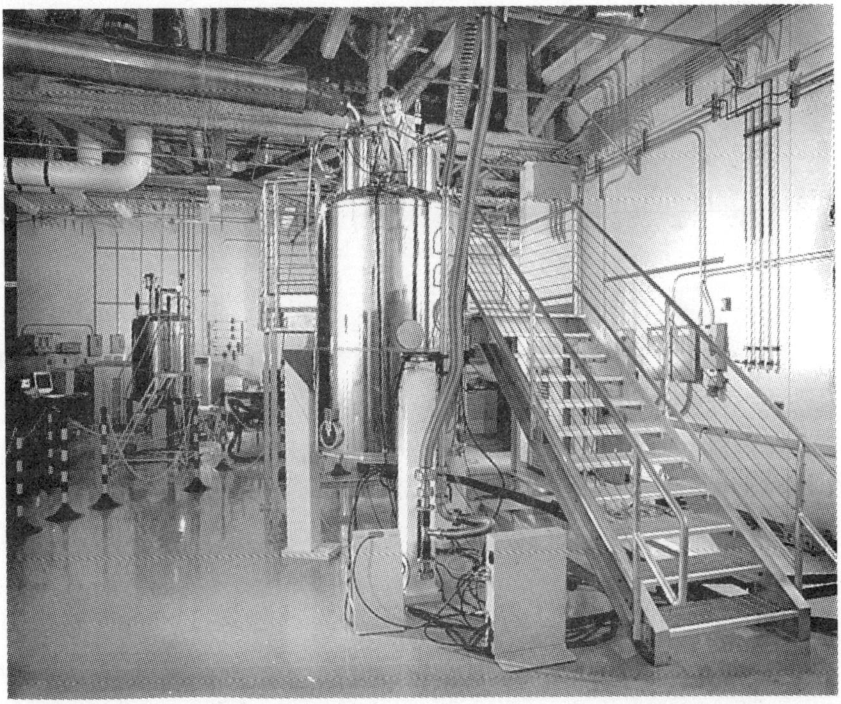

Fig. 11.8: A photograph of 800 MHz NMR spectrometer (Pacific Northwest National Laboratory instrument, photograph taken from internet)

2. Pulsed Fourier Transform (FT) Instrument

It is a more sophisticated and powerful instrument which works on the principal of single powerful excitation of all the protons present in the sample using a short burst of energy known as 'pulse' using strong magnetic field, say 2.1 Tesla for 1 – 10 μ sec burst releases 90 MHz energy. After the pulse is stopped the excited molecules start coming to ground state by loosing their energy and returning back to same spin state or relax.

Each proton when it is coming back to same spin state or relaxes, it emits electromagnetic radiation. Since many different types of protons/nuclei are present in a molecule, many different frequencies of electromagnetic radiations are emitted simultaneously. This is known as free induction decay (FID) signal. The intensity of FID decays with time as nuclei come back to their original state. Thus, FID is a combination of all frequencies emitted which are superimposed on each other and is very complex. The extraction of individual frequency of different nuclei from FID is done with the help of computer and mathematical method called Fourier transform (FT) analysis [Fig. 11.9 (a)]. These FIDs are converted to typical NMR spectra [(Fig. 11.9 (b)] using various computer programs like MestRec.

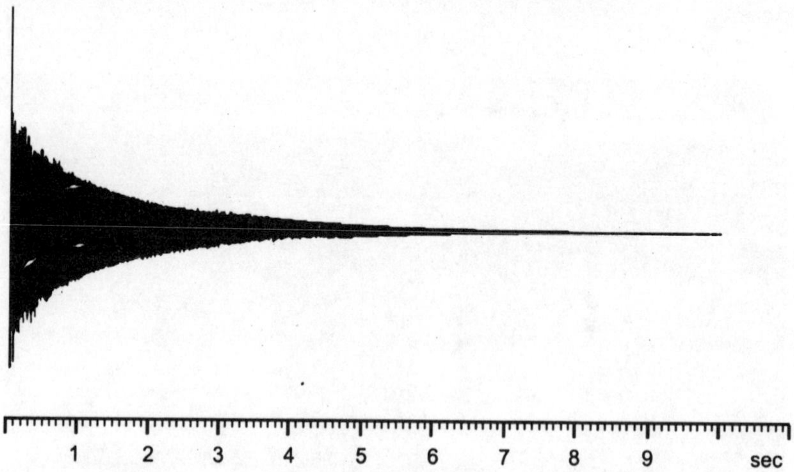

Fig. 11.9 (a)

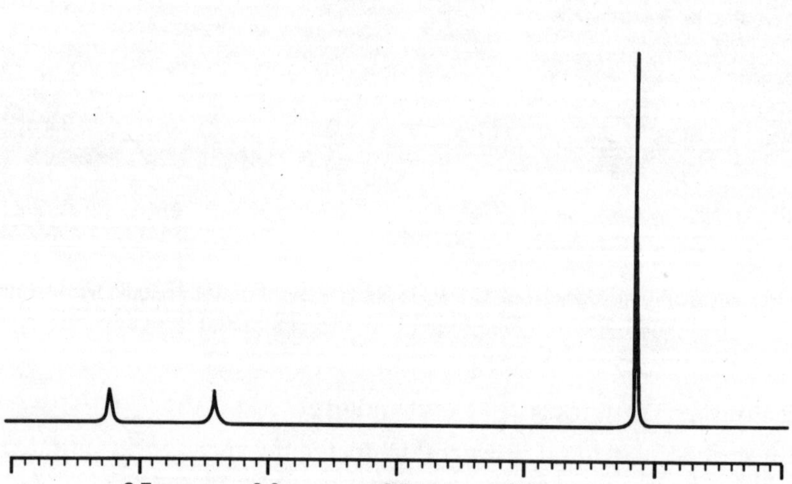

Fig. 11.9 (b)

The FT has certain advantages over CW instrumentation method. These are as follows:

- More sensitive.
- Less time is required in doing NMR.
- Very small amount of sample is required for analysis.
- Noise level is substantially reduced and signal-to-noise ratio improves as a function of square root of number of scans:

$$\frac{S}{N} = f\sqrt{n}$$

Interpretation of NMR Spectrum

The NMR spectrum appears in the form of peaks usually ranging from 0 to 12 ppm. The various protons belonging to various functional groups present in variable environment appear at different places as depicted in Fig. 11.10.

All chemically/magnetically equivalent protons appear at the same place and will give single peak, i.e. they will behave like one proton but with larger integration.

Chemically equivalent protons are those protons that have identical chemical environment, e.g. CH_3OCH_3, H_a and H_b are chemically equivalent protons, and they appear at the same place in NMR. The chemically equivalent protons behave similarly

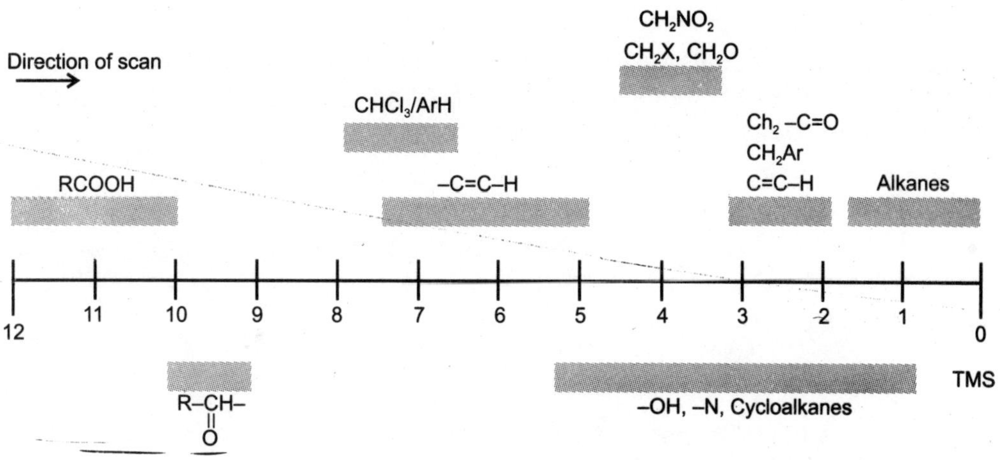

Fig. 11.10: A chart depicting protons chemical shift values

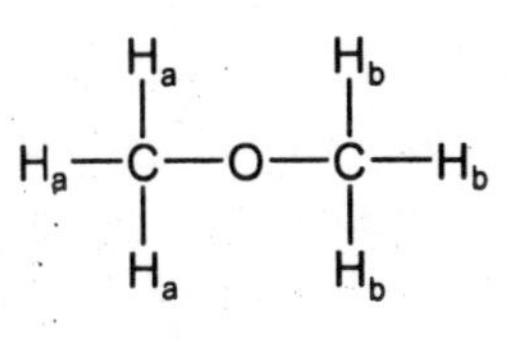

in magnetic fields thus they are called magnetically equivalent protons also, as depicted in Fig. 11.11.

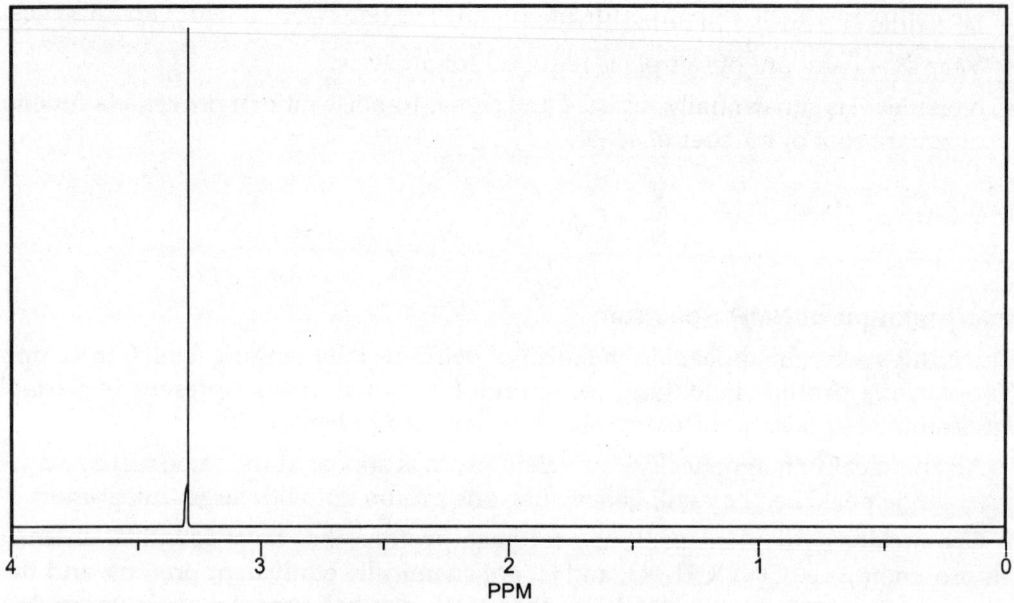

Fig. 11.11: NMR spectrum of dimethyl ether

In benzene all the protons are equivalent, therefore, there is only one peak. In CH_3OH there are two types of protons and in CH_3CH_2OH there are three types of protons, therefore, there will be two and three peaks respectively in NMR spectrum.

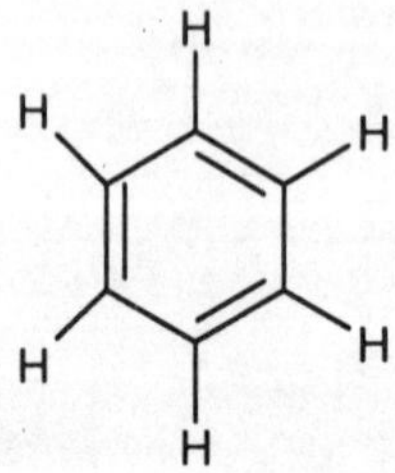

All the peaks in NMR spectrum are integrated, the value of integral can either be calculated graphically or it might be provided by the recorder. These integration values are used to determine the relative numbers of protons each peak is indicating, i.e. it gives the ratio of the number of equivalent protons in each peak.

As the ability of NMR lies in the fact that all the protons in a compound are not equivalent and, therefore, show resonance at different energy levels. The protons are different because they are surrounded by different chemical environment, i.e. different number of electron in the valence shell and different types of atoms. These differences lend them their characteristics and hence, the peak values appear at different points in NMR spectrum.

The protons which are attached to electronegative atoms like oxygen, nitrogen, halogen and sulphur are deshielded by them more strongly and hence, appear more downfield than expected.

If we compare alkanes (sp^3 hybridization), alkenes (sp^2 hybridization) and alkynes (sp hybridization); we observe that in case of alkanes where all the hydrogens are sp^3 hybridized and there are no electronegative elements or π-bonded group in vicinity, therefore, they appear from 0 to 2 ppm. Then if we think logically after alkanes towards their left first should be alkenes and then alkynes; but that is not the case. Actually while going from right to left in an NMR spectrum first will be alkanes, then alkynes and last would be alkenes.

The interchange of positions between alkenes and alkynes is attributed to magnetic anisotropy, which causes shielding effect in alkynes. The same magnetic anisotropy is responsible for the deshielding effect in case of aromatic protons. The following section explains it.

Magnetic Anisotropy

The benzene ring is a C_6H_6, closed ring, aromatic system having π electron clouds above and below the ring. When it is placed in a magnetic field, the π electron in the aromatic ring system is induced to circulate around the ring, known as ring current. The moving electron generates a magnetic field much like one generated in a loop of wire through which current is passing. The applied magnetic field becomes anisotropic (nonuniform) near the benzene molecule as this π electron generated magnetic field interferes with it (Fig. 11.12).

Thus there are three types of forces which work on benzene protons:

- The applied magnetic field
- The electrons in the valance shell around the protons
- Anisotropy generated by π-electron ring system.

The second and third forces are weaker forces as compared to applied magnetic field. But it is the anisotropic effect which gives benzene protons a chemical shift more than expected, only because the protons of benzene ring just happen to lie towards the outer side of the ring, which is the deshielding region of anisotropic field. If these protons were inside the ring, they would have been shielded by anisotropic effect. But as the protons of benzene ring are on the outer side, the amount of magnetic field experienced by them is the sum total of applied magnetic field (B_0) and the magnetic field generated by anisotropic effect. This phenomenon of experiencing increased magnetic field in comparison to applied magnetic filed is known as deshielding. This deshielding shifts the aromatic protons towards the left side in the NMR spectra, i.e. they undergo resonance at higher frequency compared to the other not deshielded or shielded protons.

The same anisotropy is responsible for the shielding of acetylene protons, which this time just happen to lie in the shielding region of anisotropic field, thus they appear more upfield than their expected position (Fig. 11.13).

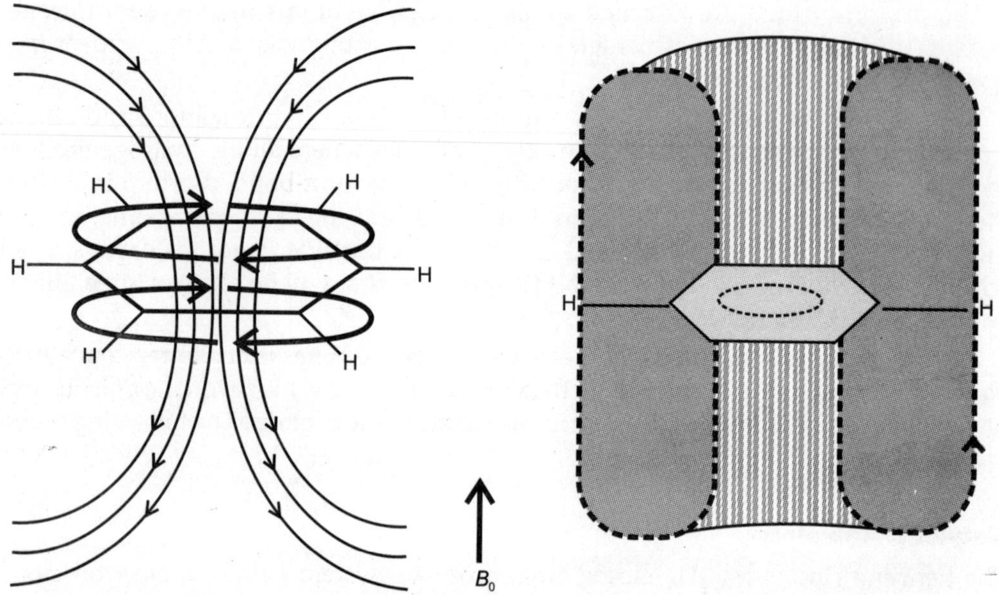

Fig. 11.12: Diamagnetic anisotropy in benzene leading to deshielding of the protons

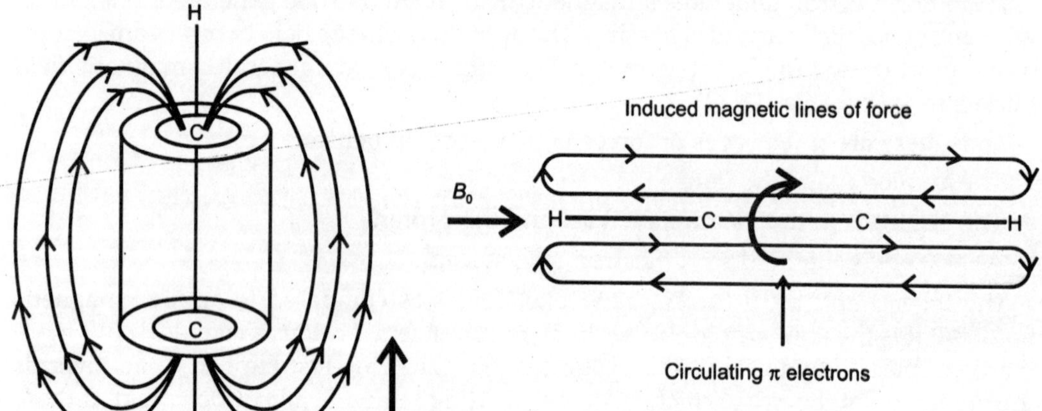

Fig. 11.13: Diamagnetic anisotropy in acetylene leading to shielding of the protons

Spin-Spin Splitting/(*n* + 1) Rule

Apart from chemical shift and value of integration another information we can get from NMR spectrum is about spin-spin splitting. In a ^{1}H-NMR spectrum all equivalent protons do not appear as a single peak, e.g. 1, 1, 2-tribromoethane has two types of equivalent protons, thus it should show two peaks in NMR spectra, but that is not the case. The actual spectrum consists of two peaks but subdivided into 3 and 2 sub peaks or splitting, integrating for one (–CH) and two ($-CH_2Br$) protons respectively.

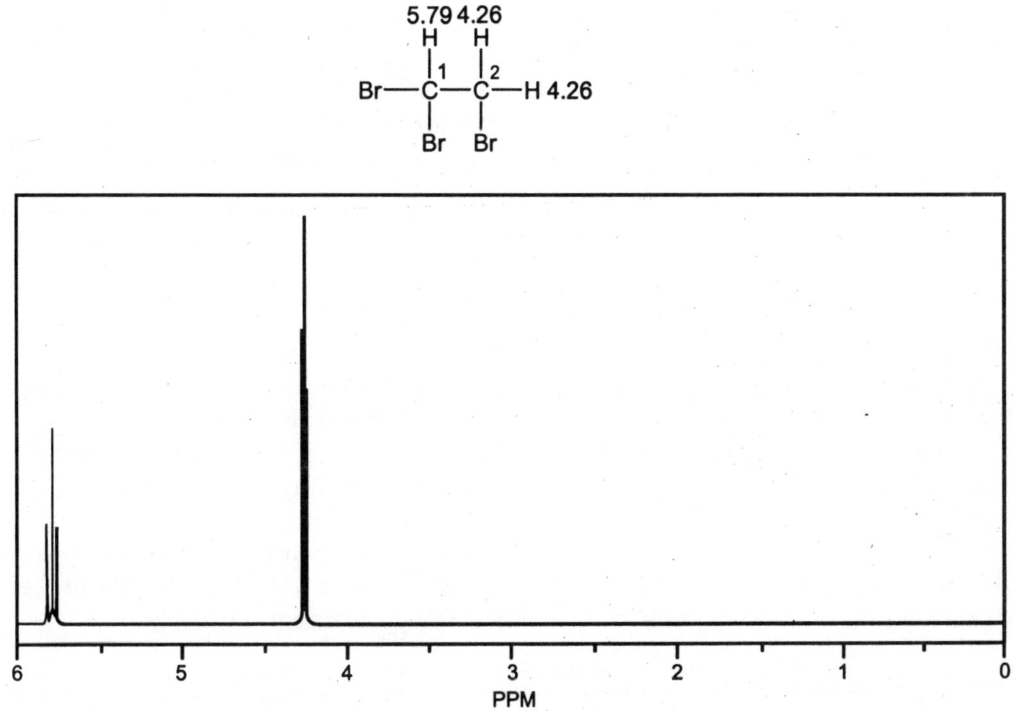

Fig. 11.14: NMR spectrum of 1, 1, 2-tribromomethane showing *n* + 1 splitting

This phenomenon of splitting of equivalent protons into $n + 1$ peaks, where n is the number of equivalent protons attached to the adjacent carbon to which the proton under consideration is attached, is called spin-spin splitting. So as per $n + 1$ rule in case of 1, 1, 2-tribromoethane; the first carbon (C_1) has two equivalent protons of methylene on the carbon next to it, therefore, $n = 2$, and hence, it will split into $2 + 1 = 3$ peaks (triplet). The methylene protons are having $n = 1$ (methane proton) therefore, the split will be $1 + 1 = 2$ peaks (doublet) (Fig. 11.14).

Spin-spin splitting occurs because the protons on the adjacent carbon can sense each other. This means that proton on adjacent carbons can shield or deshield each other, e.g. we consider a simple molecule in which only one hydrogen is attached to each carbon (Fig. 11.15).

Now H_1 while undergoing resonance in applied magnetic field is affected by H_2 (hydrogen). At the beginning the given number of molecules in a sample possess H_2 (hydrogen) with spin state $+1/2$ and $-1/2$ in equal proportion. The H_2 (hydrogen) having spin state of $+1/2$ will provide deshielding effect on H_1 as it is aligned in the same direction as that of the magnetic field B_0. Those H_2 which are having spin state of $-1/2$ will have a shielding effect on H_1 as it is aligned in the opposite direction to B_0. Therefore, half the H_1 will absorb at downfield (deshielded) and half at comparative upfield (shielded) giving two splits in a peak due to neighboring H_2. The same will be the case of H_2 because of H_1. Thus, we get both H_1 and H_2 as doublets due to each other (Fig. 11.16).

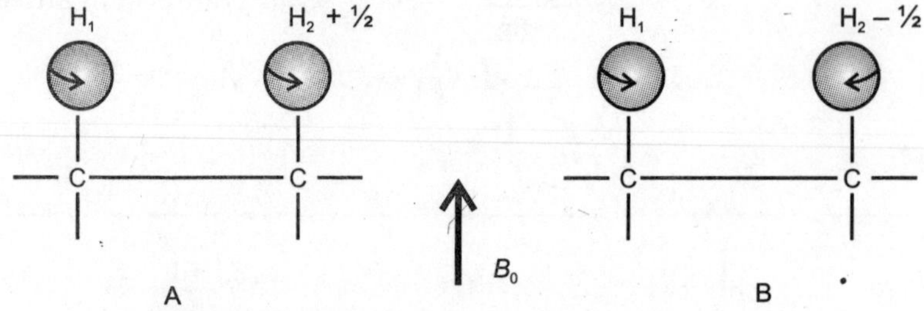

Fig. 11.15: Two different types of molecules *A* and *B*, differing in spin relationship between protons H_1 and H_2

To understand this concept further, now we will take another example of ethyl fluoride, CH_3CH_2F. This compound contains two types of chemically equivalent protons. When its NMR is taken (Fig. 11.17), it consists of two peaks splitted into triplet and quartet. The triplet peak, as now we can find out by $n + 1$ rule, will be of the proton which is having two equivalent protons attached to the adjacent carbon, hence it is a peak of $-CH_3$ protons. The other peak which is a quartet is of $-CH_2$ protons, in which splitting has taken place because of neighboring methyl protons. The numbers of protons present in each peak are calculated using the integration value.

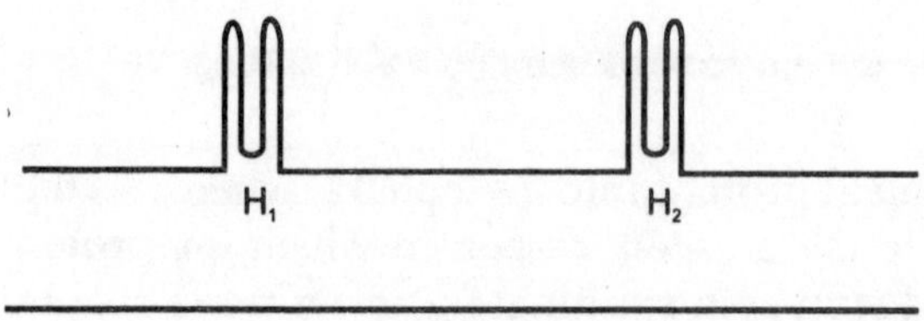

Fig. 11.16

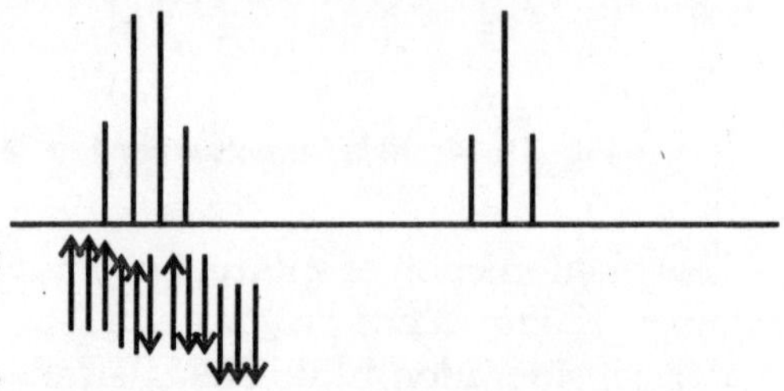

Fig. 11.17: The splitting pattern of ethyl fluoride protons

Coupling Constant

Coupling constant is a constant which quantifies the amount by which peaks spilt. For example, if there is an ortho, meta or para coupling between the protons in an aromatic system the value of J_0, J_p and J_m will be same in all systems. Hence, by calculating 'J' value we can estimate what kind of coupling is taking place. It helps in determining the structure of an unknown compound by letting us know whether the compound is *cis* or *trans* or whether it is having protons at *ortho*, *meta* or *para* position or any other type of proton.

The same example of ethyl fluoride can be considered to explain the coupling constant. The coupling constant of quartet and triplet splitting obtained in that NMR can be calculated. The quartet can be divided into three equal J values and triplet into 2 Js. To calculate the J value we should take the exact d values of the two peaks whose J value is to be calculated. Subtract the two values (higher one from the lower one) and divide it by the MHz on which the instrument was operated, e.g. 60, 120, 300, etc.

$$J = \frac{\delta_1 - \delta_2}{\text{MHz}}$$

Some common J values

$$J_{cis} = 5-10$$
$$J_{trans} = 10-17$$
$$J_p = 0-1$$
$$J_m = 1-3$$
$$J_o = 6-10$$

The coupling constants of a group of protons that split one another must be identical.

^{1}H–NMR of Some Compounds

1. **C_2H_5OH** (Fig. 11.18).

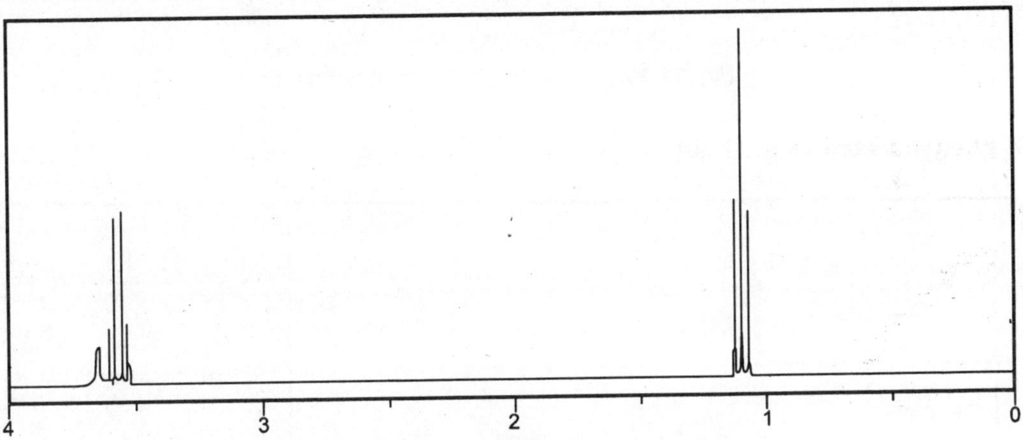

Fig. 11.18: ^{1}H-NMR spectrum of ethanol

^{1}H–NMR (ppm rel. to TMS)

Node	Shift
OH	3.65 (triplet, because of $-CH_2$ protons)
CH_2	3.57 (multiplet, because of OH and $-CH_2$ protons)
CH_3	1.10 (triplet, because of $-CH_2$ protons)

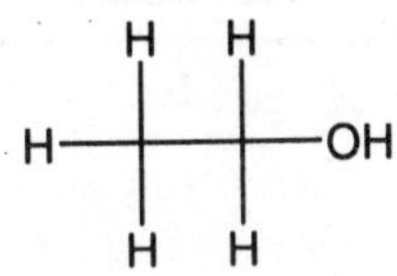

2. **$C_6H_5NH_2$** (Fig. 11.19)

^{1}H–NMR (ppm rel. to TMS)

Node	Shift
NH_2	6.27 (triplet)
CH	6.63 (doublet)
CH	6.63 (doublet)
CH	7.20 (triplet)
CH	7.20 (triplet)
CH	6.81 (triplet)

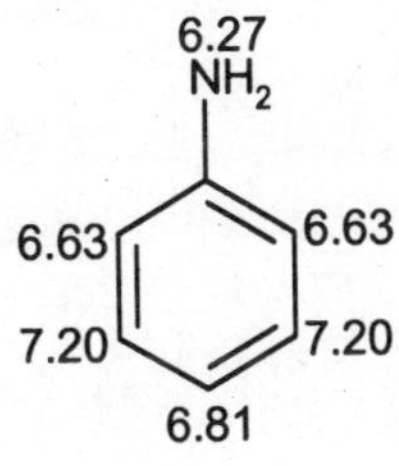

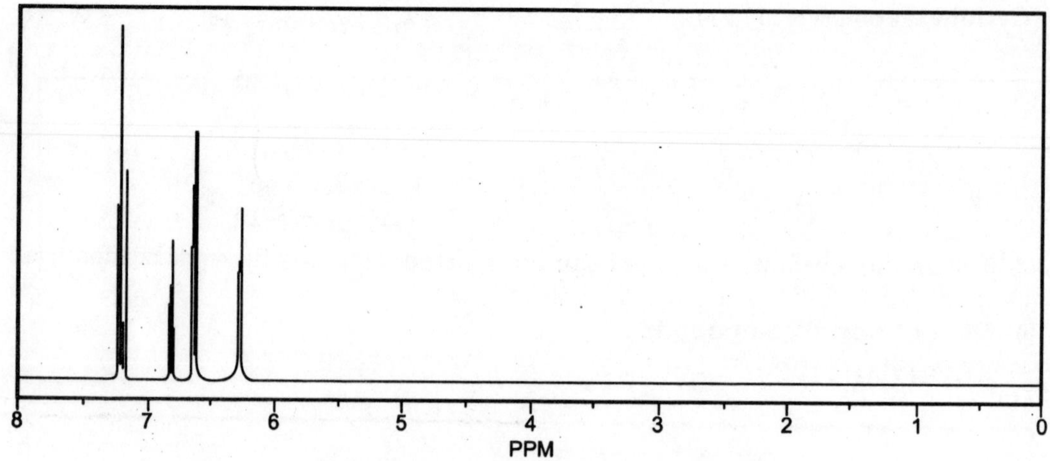

Fig. 11.19: ^{1}H–NMR spectrum of aniline

3. **Phenyl acetate** (Fig. 11.20)

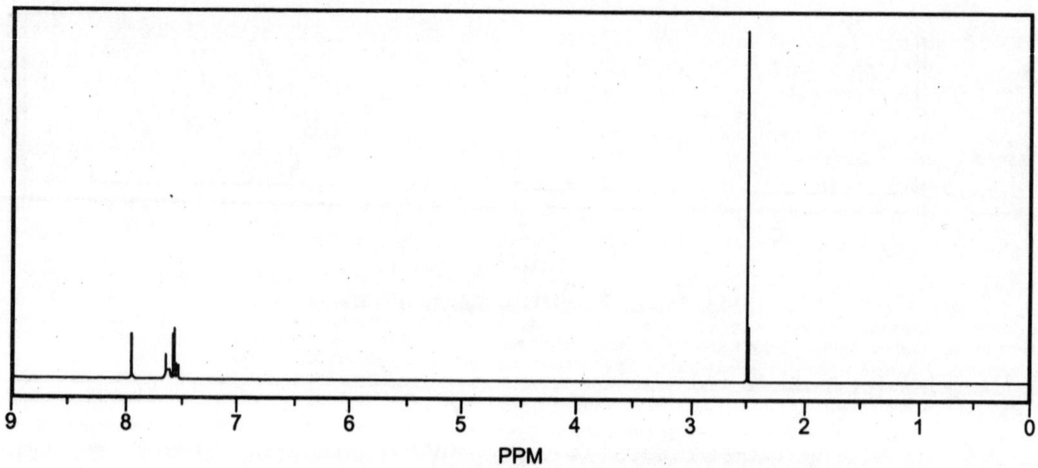

Fig. 11.20: ^{1}H–NMR spectrum of phenyl acetate

^{1}H–NMR (ppm rel. to TMS)

Node	Shift
CH	7.94
CH	7.94
CH	7.56
CH	7.56
CH	7.64
CH_3	2.50

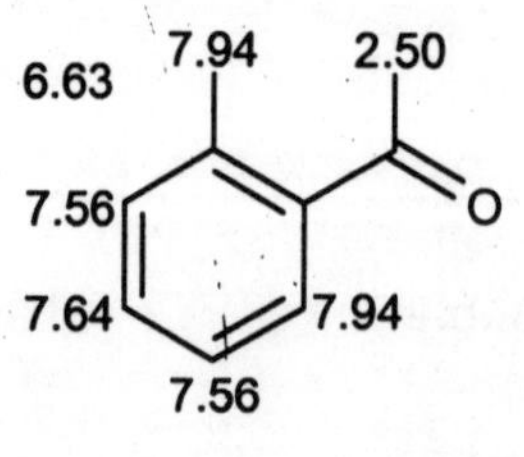

4. **Cyclohexanone** (Fig. 11.21)

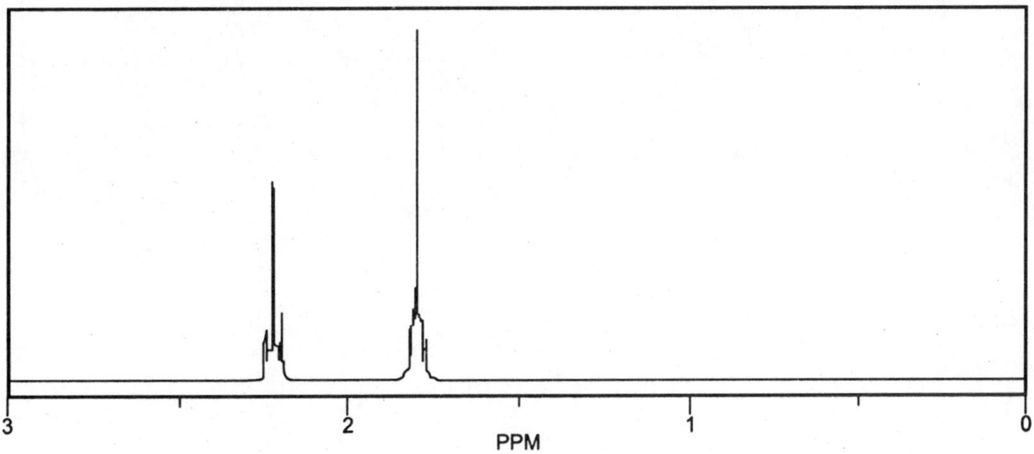

Fig. 11.21: ^{1}H–NMR spectrum of cyclohexanone

^{1}H–NMR (ppm rel. to TMS)

Node	Shift
CH_2	2.22
CH_2	2.22
CH_2	1.80
CH_2	1.80
CH_2	1.80

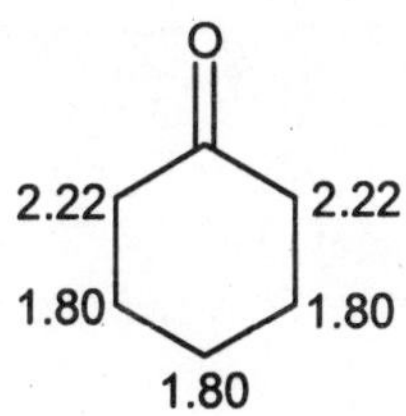

BIBLIOGRAPHY

1. Gunther H, in *NMR* 2nd edn., John Wiley and Sons, New York, 1995.
2. Pavia DL, Lampman GM, Kriz GS., in *Introduction to Spectroscopy*, 3rd edn., Brooks/Cole, Thompson, USA, 2001.
3. Silverstein RM, Webster FX, in *Spectrometric Identification of Organic Compounds*, 6th edn., John Wiley and Sons, New York, 1998.

12 Combinatorial Chemistry and High Throughput Screening

COMBINATORIAL CHEMISTRY

Introduction

Finding a novel drug is a complex process. Historically, the main source of biologically active compounds used in drug discovery programs has been natural products, isolated from plants, animals or fermentation sources. Then came the synthetic approach, where these active molecules were tried to synthesize in lab using conventional (one-molecule-at-a-time in solution phase) methods. Their structural modification was done to obtain therapeutically better entities.

Combinatorial chemistry is one of the important relatively newer synthetic methodologies developed to reduce the time and costs associated with producing effective and competitive new drugs. In a way combinatorial chemistry has revolutionized approaches to discovering promising new lead molecules not only for drugs, but also more recently for making catalysts and many other target molecules. The rapidly evolving technology of combi-chemistry makes it possible to produce compound libraries to be screened for novel biological activities. Thus, this powerful new technology has helped the pharmaceutical companies to find new drug candidates quickly, save significant money in preclinical development costs and ultimately change their fundamental approach to drug discovery.

History

The origins of combinatorial chemistry can be traced back to 1963, when biochemistry Professor R. Bruce Merrifield of Rockefeller University, New York, developed a way to make peptides by solid-phase synthesis. But the field in its modern dimensions only began to take shape in the 1980s, when research scientist H. Mario Geysen, developed a technique to synthesize arrays of peptides on pin-shaped solid supports and Houghten developed a technique for creating peptide libraries in tiny mesh 'tea bags' by solid-phase parallel synthesis.

Although peptide and oligonucleotide libraries are still very much of interest, the combinatorial field has moved towards libraries of drug-like small organic molecules. In the early 1990s, J.A. Ellman and S.H. DeWitt independently worked out some of the earliest techniques for producing small-molecule libraries. Some of the success stories using combinatorial chemistry are of the molecules developed by Trega Biosciences, San Diego, which is in clinical trials for pain and asthma; Magainin Pharmaceuticals and Merck also have compounds in clinical trials that were clearly based on early combinatorial approaches; an orally active thrombin inhibitor developed by T.R. Webb is in use now.

Principle and Methodology

Traditional approaches to synthesize individual molecules using solution phase methods have been and continue to be very successful, allowing chemists to synthesize molecules of great complexity. However, this concept of synthesizing one molecule after another has its limitations; using this approach a medicinal chemist is expected to synthesize around 100 molecules in a year. Considering the infinitesimally small number of molecules that make it to the market, classical methods of drug discovery-involving purification of intermediate compounds using methods such as extraction and chromatography are, therefore, lengthy and expensive.

Combinatorial chemistry, on the other hand, uses solid support to carry out the reaction. The reactants are allowed to pass through a column of solid packing material on which the reaction takes place. The reaction is allowed to proceed to completion by using excess amounts of reagents, which can simply be washed away in the end. The goal of solid phase chemistry is to overcome the need for labor-intensive purification by using filtration as sole method of purification.

The purpose of combinatorial chemistry is twofolds. First, to assemble as quickly as possible compounds for screening, with the objective of finding a 'lead' compound possessing desired properties. Usually, this involves synthesis of a large number of molecules in very small quantities. Secondly, once a 'lead' has been found, combinatorial chemistry can be used to synthesize analogues to improve the potency, efficacy of a compound as potential drug; or selectivity of the compound as catalyst or any other target product.

The solid phase used in most of the combinatorial reaction is generally a resin insoluble polymer that swells in the presence of the reaction solvent, but which is inert to reaction conditions. The most widely used support is polystyrene, which is cross-linked with 1 percent divinyl benzene to give the polymer structural rigidity and to tender it insoluble. Another common solid support is Tentagel resin, which consists of polyethylene glycol attached to polystyrene through an ether linker (Fig. 12.1). This resin is particularly useful for the reactions which take place in water,

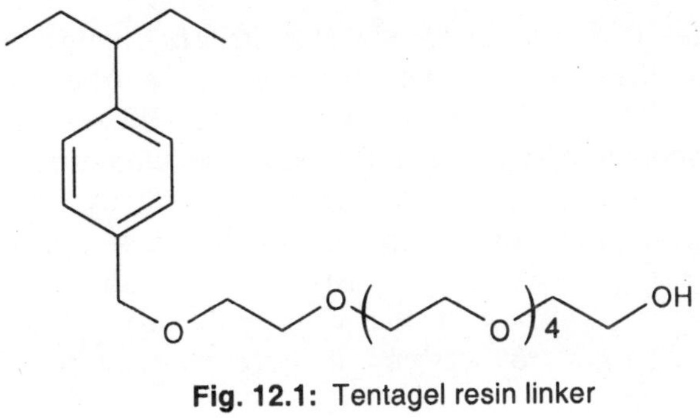

Fig. 12.1: Tentagel resin linker

like biotransformations. The hydrophilic nature of the support allows solvation to occur in aqueous solvent mixtures.

Linker is another crucial element in the solid phase synthesis. It acts as a link to attach the organic molecule to the polymeric support. Designing of linkers is a challenging area of research for the scientists working in the field of combinatorial chemistry, their modifications have greatly extended the combinatorial chemists arsenal. Like protecting group in organic synthesis, the linker must survive the conditions of the synthesis, and be readily detachable from resin without destroying the synthesized molecules once the reaction is complete.

Monitoring the progress of reaction on solid supports is also challenging. One option is to cleave quantities of resin at various intervals during the reaction and use standard analytical methods to assess the amounts of intermediates and/or products formed. However, there are other methods like chemical tests (Kaiser test for peptide coupling), FTIR, MS, NMR that are more convenient and less time consuming.

At a very basic level solid phase reactions can be carried out using conventional glassware. The specific apparatus has been designed primarily to ease the holding of multiple reaction vessels and to aid work up of many parallel reactions, e.g. designing of polypropylene syringe complete with sinter disk for filtering and washing the products directly after the reaction takes place in the same vessel. The next step can be proceeded by simply adding more reagents and solvents in this vessel. Reactions in the syringe are mechanically shaken rather than stirred, helping to prevent mechanical degradation of the resin, which might occur with stirrer bead. Apart from this now many other highly sophisticated fully automated synthesizers are available which automatically carry out the tedious resin filtration and washing. These machines also allow the chemists to carry out a full range of solution and solid phase synthetic manipulations, controlled through software.

After synthesis the next step is the solvent removal using efficient heated vacuum centrifuges, which evaporates corrosive solvents. The final step, that is the purification and analysis of results is also automated which most of the times uses LC-MS as both an analytical tool and in a preparative manner.

Approaches to Combinatorial Chemistry

The traditional drug design and combinatorial chemistry both rely on organic synthesis methodologies. The difference between the two lies in the scope—instead of synthesizing a single compound, combinatorial chemistry exploits automation and miniaturization of reactions to synthesize large libraries of compounds. But because large libraries do not produce active compounds independently, scientists also need a straightforward way to find the active components within these enormous populations. Thus, combinatorial organic synthesis (COS) is not random, but by using sets of chemical 'building blocks' to form a diverse set of molecular entities either spatially, through chemical encoding, or by systematic, successive synthesis and biological evaluation (deconvolution).

There are four common approaches to COS:

- ***Arrayed synthesis:*** In arrayed, spatially addressable synthesis, building blocks are reacted systematically in individual reaction wells or positions to form separated 'discrete molecules'. Active compounds are identified by their location on the grid. One such type of arrayed synthesis is *mix and split synthesis/divide couple recombine* which involves distributing a pool of resin beads into separate reaction vessel, each with single different reactant or building block. This makes sure that each bead comes in contact with one reactant and avoids competition between slow and fast reactions, which occurs in conventional one-pot combinatorial chemistry procedures, e.g. at the start of the reaction the resin is divided into three equal portions (Fig. 12.2). Each of this portion is then reacted individually with a building block X_1, X_2 and X_3. After the reaction is complete, the beads are filtered and washed. The resulting resins are mixed to randomize the solid supported compounds X_1, X_2 and X_3. These are then split again into three equal portions and treated with building blocks Y_1, Y_2 and Y_3, to give a total of nine products, as three mixtures of three compounds. Repeating this cycle can result in a very large number of compounds.

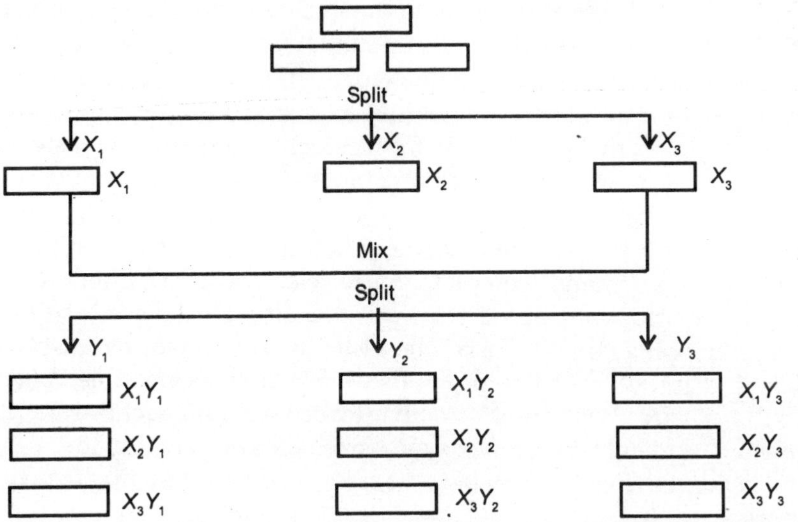

Fig. 12.2: The mix and split scheme for the synthesis of nine compounds for a library

- ***Encoded mixture synthesis:*** This technique uses nucleotide, peptide, or other types of more inert chemical tags to identify each compound.
- ***Deconvolution synthesis:*** During deconvolution, a series of compound mixtures is synthesized combinatorially, each time fixing some specific structural feature. Each mixture is assayed as a mixture and the most active combination is pursued. Further rounds systematically fix other structural features until a manageable number of discrete structures can be synthesized and screened. Scientists working with peptides, for example, can use deconvolution to optimize, or locate, the most active peptide sequence from millions of possibilities.

- *Solution phase:* Ideal reactions for the solution synthesis are those that are kinetically and thermodynamically favored, are tolerant to a range of functionality and have a broad range of tolerance towards the reactants. The capture resin and extraction procedures are normally used for preliminary purification. Derivatization of functionalized scaffolds and multi-component condensation reaction are the common methods used to synthesize the solution phase libraries.

Managing Combinatorial Chemistry Libraries

As with traditional drug design, the ability to integrate different types of chemical and biological information is crucial to combinatorial chemistry techniques. Once built, combinatorial libraries produce unprecedented amounts of information. Reaction histories for each compound must be traceable. Scientists need to integrate screening results and biological data with structural information. The combinatorial libraries and their corresponding data is essential to cost-effective research and development.

Enumeration of a parent library is an important aspect as it enables the researcher to produce structural representations of child libraries, or discrete compounds within the library. *Enumeration* is the process of automatically generating either subgeneric or fully specified structures (individual compounds) from a generic structure.

In combinatorial chemistry, the ability to manage the building blocks that make up the libraries is just as important as the ability to manage libraries themselves. The building block structures make it possible for researchers to gain new insight into the biological effectiveness of individual building blocks by tracking their success across libraries and screens.

Combinatorial chemistry is a promising new field that stands to revolutionize the chemical industry, and demands completely new scientific information management solutions. It is a technologically advanced way of finding a needle in a haystack. The whole idea of employing combinatorial chemistry is to remove the guesswork and instead create and test as many compounds or mixtures as possible, *logically* and *systematically*, to obtain a viable set of active leads. With an orchestrate planning, building, screening, and interpretation of synthesized libraries, combinatorial chemistry can be helpful in minimizing the time and cost associated with bringing new molecular entities to market.

HIGH THROUGHPUT SCREENING

Rate of synthesis of new compounds, using combinatorial approach or conventional method has led to a tremendous increase in the volume of new compound library both for peptides and organic compounds. Thus, there is a need for equally efficient screening system for these entities. High-Throughput Screening or HTS allows us to quickly conduct millions of biochemical, genetic or pharmacological tests, using robotics, data processing and control software, liquid handling devices, and sensitive detectors. Through this process one can rapidly identify active compounds, antibodies or genes which modulate a particular biomolecular pathway. The results of these experiments provide starting points for drug design and for understanding the interaction or role of a particular biochemical process in biology. Hence, HTS can be employed for both pharmacodynamic and pharmacokinetic studies.

HTS screens a library of candidate compounds using an assay done in a fully automated manner. An assay is a test for specific activity: usually inhibition or stimulation of a biochemical or biological mechanism. Typical HTS screening libraries also known as 'decks' can contain from 100,000 to more than 2,000,000 compounds. The compounds which are identified from such screenings are termed as *HIT* a molecule with confirmed activity from primary HTS assay with good profile in secondary assay and having a confirmed structutre; and *Lead* a HIT series for which the structure activity relationship is shown and activities demonstrated *in vitro* and *in vivo*.

Methodology

The key labware or testing vessel of HTS is the microtiter plate, which is a small container, usually disposable and made of plastic, which features a grid of small, open divot called well. Modern microplates for HTS generally have either 384, 1536, or 3456 wells. These are all multiples of 96, reflecting the original 96 well microplate with 8 × 129 mm spaced wells. Most of the wells contain experimentally useful matter, often an aqueous solution of dimethyl sulfoxide (DMSO) and some other chemical compound which is different for each well across the plate. Some wells may be used as optional experimental controls.

To prepare for an assay, each well of the plate is filled with a specific concentration of the compounds to be tested and some biological entity on which the experiment is to be conducted, such as a protein, some cells, or an animal embryo. After addition it is left for incubation for some time to allow the biological matter to absorb, bind to, or otherwise react (or fail to react) with the compounds in the wells. Then the measurements are taken across all the plates' wells, either manually for example using microscopy to seek changes or defects in embryonic development caused by the wells' compounds; or by a machine such as shining polarized light on them and measuring reflectivity, which can be an indication of protein binding. In each case, the machine outputs the result of each experiment as a grid of numeric values, with each number pertaining to the value obtained from a single well. For estimation of the assay HTS generally uses luminescence-based detection. Various fluorescence techniques like Fluorescence Anisotropy (FA), Fluroscence Correlation Spectroscopy (FCS), Fluorescence Intensity (FI), Fluorescence Lifetime Imaging Spectroscopy (FLIM), Fluorescence Resonance Energy Transfer (FRET), Total Internal Reflection Fluorescence (TIRF) and Time Resolved Resonance Anisotropy (TRRA) are used. Along with that LC-MS and LC-NMR are also used at times, e.g in metabolic or absorption studies. A high-capacity analysis machine can measure dozens of plates in the span of a few minutes generating thousands of experimental datapoints very quickly.

Depending on the results of this first assay, follow up assays can be performed within the same screen by picking the liquid from the source wells that gave interesting results (known as 'hits') into new assay plates, and then re-running the experiment to collect further data on this narrowed set, confirming and refining observations.

A screening facility typically contains a library of *stock plates,* whose contents are carefully catalogued, and each of which may have been created by the lab or obtained from a commercial source. These stock plates themselves are not directly used in experiments; instead, separate *assay plates* are created as needed. An assay plate is simply a copy of a stock plate, created by pipetting a small amount of liquid (often measured in nanoliters) from the wells of a stock plate to the corresponding wells of a completely empty plate.

Automation is an important factor in HTS's usefulness. Typically, an integrated robotic system consists of automated transport of assay microplates from one station to another for sample and reagent addition, mixing, incubation, and finally readout or detection. An HTS system can usually prepare, incubate, and analyze many plates simultaneously, further speeding the data collection process. HTS robots currently exist which can test up to 100,000 compounds per day. The uHTS or ultra high throughput screening system is the technique employed for the screening systems, which can be used to screen more than 100,000 compounds per day.

Unique distributions of compounds across one or many plates can be employed either to increase the number of assays per plate, or to reduce the variance of assay results, or both. The simplifying assumption made in this approach is that any *'N'* compounds in the same well will not typically interact with each other, or the assay target, in a manner that fundamentally changes the ability of the assay to detect true hits. For example, imagine a plate where compound *X* is in wells 1–2–3, compound *Y* is in wells 2–3–4, and compound *Z* is in wells 3–4–5. In an assay of this plate against a given target, a hit in wells 3, 4, and 5 would indicate that compound *Z* is the most active agent, while also providing three values of compound *Z*'s efficacy against the specified target. When employed commercially, this approach uses combinations in which no two compounds ever share more than one well, to reduce the (second-order) possibility of interference between pairs of compounds being screened.

HTS is a relatively recent innovation, made feasible through advances in automation and high-speed computer technology. It still takes a highly specialized and expensive screening lab to run an HTS operation, thus small-to-moderately sized research institution should use the services of an existing HTS facility rather than set up one for itself.

BIBLIOGRAPHY

1. Appell K, Baldwin JJ, Egan WJ, Combinatorial Chemistry and High throughput screening in drug discovery and development. In: *Handbook of Modern Pharmaceutical Analysis.* Ahuja S and Scypinski S, Ed., Academic Press, an Imprint of Elsevier, San Diego, California, 2005, p-23–56..
2. Dolle RE, Nelson K H Jr, J Comb. Chem., 1999, 1, 235–82
3. G Bhalay, Chemistry in Britain, 1999, March, 25–28.
4. http://www.netsci.org/Science/Combichem/feature02.html.
5. In *Combonatorial Chemistry: Synthesis, Analysis,* Gunther Jung, ed., Wiley-VCH, 1999.
6. Suto MJ, Curr. Opin. Drug Disc. Dev., 1999, 2: 377–84.

13 Statistical Analysis of Bioequivalence Study and Clinical Trials

INTRODUCTION

Statistical analysis is an essential part of clinical trials. Clinical studies are very expensive, so proper planning is extremely essential to make these studies meet their objectives. Clinical trial is a specialized field with its own terminology.

Some Important Terms

Controlled study: A controlled study is one in which control groups are included to avoid bias. Controls can be pharmacologically active ingredients or placebo.

Placebo effect: Human beings can respond to stimuli as a result of their psychology. Sometimes, a patient may get well just by believing that he has been on drugs. This is known as placebo effect.

Blinding: To avoid bias, the patients and the observers are kept ignorant about the nature of the treatment. In double blind technique, both patients and doctors are kept unaware. In single blind technique, only the subjects are kept unaware.

Precision: Lesser the variability, greater is the precision. Because of the biological variation between the patients, data obtained from the clinical studies vary widely. Precision is improved by increasing the number of patients enrolled for a study. If the effects observed among the members of a group are highly variable, it raises the question of reliability of drug effect. Use of baseline measurement or use of a crossover design can increase precision. Blocking is another way to increase precision. In this design, patients are matched for characteristics that are likely to exert some influence on drug effects. If a drug has high volume of distribution, the result is likely to be affected by the body weight variations. In such cases, greater control of body weight is to be exercised. To balance the experimental groups, if a man of 60 kg is assigned to one group, another person of similar weight is to be assigned to other group.

Symmetry: This indicates equality of the treatment. Equal number of patients in each group, equal number of observations per patient or equality in their characteristics (age, sex, etc.) ensures symmetry of an experiment.

Randomization: Patients are assigned to groups according to a particular design. Subjects are numbered and then according to the randomization blocks (Appendix 8) they are assigned to one or the other group.

Intent to treat: Often some of the members who take part in clinical trials are unable to complete the study. Subjects may be disqualified for various reasons, e.g. protocol violations or noncompliance of dosage regimen. Data obtained from such subjects are important with respect to safety and adverse drug reactions. In 'Intent to treat' analysis, efficacy data are analyzed including these people.

DESIGNS USED IN CLINICAL TRIAL

Parallel design: In parallel design, two or more groups can be compared simultaneously and each group has different subjects. Subjects are allocated to groups according to randomization procedure. Normally, subjects are numbered consecutively. In a comparison of two groups, half of the subjects are coded with odd numbers and the other half with even numbers. Now if there are 40 patients, a block of 8 will be suitable. Column-wise numbers of the blocks are read and odd numbered subjects are assigned to one block and even numbered ones in the other group. Parallel design saves time because all the patients receive treatment at the same time. However, use of a control group is essential. Consideration should be given in the following points.

The Objective

First, the objective of the experiment must be declared. Depending upon this objective the treatment and controls are decided. For example, if the objective of the test is to prove the efficacy of a new molecule, the new molecule should be compared against a placebo. On the other hand, if it is desired to prove that the new drug is better than the existing drug, a standard drug is to be used.

Subjects

Before exposing the subjects to the treatment, the baseline values of the parameters to be estimated (BP, blood sugar, etc.) are recorded. Baseline averages of the two treatment groups should be tested by conventional t test. The result of this test, if not significantly different, assumes that the groups are comparable.

$$t = \frac{\bar{X}_1 - \bar{X}_2}{S_p \sqrt{\frac{1}{N_1} + \frac{1}{N_2}}}$$

Here, $\bar{X}_1$ and $\bar{X}_2$ represent averaged baseline values of the two groups, S_p is the common standard deviation, N_1 and N_2 are the numbers of subjects in each group.

If baseline values are significantly different, the test becomes more complicated (covariance analysis, ratio of response to baseline, etc.).

Then the treatments are done and the observations are noted. If differences from baseline are used as benchmark for comparison of the treatment groups, the variability of the measurement can be reduced. The analysis of the treatment-results is carried according to one-way ANOVA.

Crossover Designs and Bioavailability/Bioequivalence Studies

This design is mostly used in bioavailability or bioequivalence studies. Since each patient acts as his control, inter-individual variation does not exist and results are more accurate. However, there is always a chance of carryover effect from the earlier treatment and proper washout period should be incorporated between the treatments.

Usually, two treatments are compared by this method. The order of the treatment is randomized and patients take the treatments in turn.

The crossover design is a type of Latin square design. In a Latin square design, the number of treatments equals the number of patients. So theoretically, in the comparison of two drugs *A* and *B*, two patients will be sufficient. In the first period, first patient will take drug *A* and second patient drug *B*. After the washout period, second patient will take drug *A* and first patient drug *B*. In this way, each of the drugs gets tested on each of the patients. If the effect of the drug is influenced by time or environment, the effect is nullified because the drug gets equal exposure to environmental factors.

To be statistically validated, clinical trials need large number of data. Latin square is repeated several times to include sufficient patients.

Disadvantages

Every design has its limitations. Some disadvantages are associated with crossover designs too.

Crossover design takes longer time compared to parallel design.

If the number of patients enrolled is less, missing datum is a serious problem. If one person carries out the testing of first drug but not the second, the data of the first drug becomes unusable.

Management of the experiment is difficult.

There is a possibility of carryover or residual effect.

Studies can be affected by uncontrolled factors such as psychological status of the patients as well as external factors like weather, clinical setting, etc. But in spite of all these difficulties, the crossover design is ideally suited for bioavailability studies.

Study design: Typically two period crossovers with single dose are carried out to study the bioequivalence. With multiple dose study, blood samples are taken after the drug concentration attains the steady state level. To avoid the carryover effect, a washout period of seven half-lives is recommended. Usually, the drugs tested are of similar nature and the carryover effects are often cancelled out as both the drugs have similar carryover effect. A differential carryover effect, i.e. two formulations having different types of carryover makes the analysis difficult.

For example, let us assume two brands of a drug are being compared. The brands are defined *A* and *B*. Consideration should be given in the following points.

Objective

First, the objective of the study is defined and a null hypothesis is stated.

Enrollment of Volunteers

Subjects are selected according to predefined guidelines and divided into two groups. The type of the subjects chosen for a study depends on the objective of the study. The number of subjects should be enough to have the result statistically validated.

Order of Treatment

Half of the subjects are administered the drug in one order and the other half in reverse order. For example, in the first phase, half of the subjects receive the brand *A* while the other half receive the brand *B*. In the second phase, the treatment order is reversed.

Sample Withdrawal

Blood samples are withdrawn at suitable intervals. The timing of the sampling is decided by the nature of the drug. Drugs having long half-life usually have prolonged intervals between sampling whereas drugs of short half-life or high absorption rate constant may have shorter intervals between sampling. A washout period is allowed in between two phases of study. During this period, the concentration of the first administered drug decreases and subjects go back to base level conditions. Next, the alternative product (i.e. the product in the next sequence) is administered and blood levels are determined.

Analysis

The results of the experiments are analyzed statistically. Errors may be incorporated in the study during designing as well as sample estimation. It may so happen that on a particular day the results are on the higher side due to visual error of an operator or some unknown environmental factors. To avoid such errors, the same operator should assay both the samples obtained from a particular subject, so that errors if any, get cancelled on subtraction. Usually, samples are blinded (operator does not know whether he is assaying the samples of *A* or *B*) but assessment is done in chronological order (sample withdrawn at second hour is assayed after the sample of first hour). Results are analyzed to estimate C_{max}, t_{max} and AUC.

To get the values for $AUC_{0-\infty}$, sampling needs to be done for a very long time, till the time, body is totally free of drug. But measuring instruments have their limits and concentration below a certain value cannot be estimated accurately. To solve such problems mathematical predictions are used.

Once the absorption and distribution phase is over, most of the drugs follow a monoexponential elimination pattern, governed by their overall elimination rate constant.

It is customary to determine the concentration up to 2–3 half-lives and thereafter extrapolate the log linear portion of the plasma concentration-time data to obtain the *AUC* of the terminal phase.

$$AUC_{0-\infty} = AUC_{0-t} + AUC_{t-\infty} \qquad \text{(Eq. 13.1)}$$

The value of the terminal fraction , i.e. $AUC_{t-\alpha}$ is obtained by using equation.

$$AUC_{t-\infty} = \frac{C_t}{K_E} \qquad \text{(Eq. 13.2)}$$

Where C_t represents the concentration at any time t in the terminal phase of plasma concentration-time plot (the fraction guided by elimination rate constant only) K_E = the overall elimination constant.

Comparison

Bioavailability is actually a ratio of two AUCs. The denominator represents the area of the standard formulation. Both numerator and denominator can vary but denominator is usually treated as fixed. Usually, log values of the AUCs are used rather than untransformed values.

Factors affecting Outcome of a Bioavailability/Bioequivalence Study

Let us assume two drugs *A* and *B* are being compared. Patients are divided into two groups and drugs are administered in two sequences. In the first sequence patients in group 1 take drug *A* and patients of group 2 take drug *B*. The reverse pattern is followed in the second sequence (Table 13.1). Let us assume the drug effects by intensity and let the actual intensity of drug *A* be 6 and drug *B* be 4.

Table13.1: Scheme of drug administration in 2-drug Latin square design

Sequence of administration	*Period 1*	*Period 2*
Sequence 1	*A*	*B*
Sequence 2	*B*	*A*

If the results are unaffected by time and environmental factors, data will reflect the true effect of both the drugs and results will be similar as Table 13.2.

Table 13.2: Illustration of bioequivalence data unaffected by environment and carryover

Sequence of administration	*Period 1*	*Period 2*
Sequence 1	$A = 6$	$B = 4$
Sequence 2	$B = 4$	$A = 6$

The computations in such cases are easy.

The sequence × period interaction is the treatment effect. In other words, it is the difference of effects in two sequences.

$$\text{Treatment effect } (A - B) = \frac{1}{2}\ [(A - B)_{seq-1} - (B - A)_{seq-2}]$$

$$\frac{[(6-4)-(4-6)]}{2} = 2$$

Simply stated, the average effect of

$$A = \frac{6+6}{2} = 6$$

Similarly, the effect $$B = \frac{4+4}{2} = 4$$

Average difference between A and B is $6 - 4 = 2$.

Assuming B as the standard drug, the ratio of

$$\frac{A}{B} = \frac{6}{4} = 1.5$$

The log ratio limit would be 0.8.

However, the calculation of data in a real-life bioavailability study is not so simple. The results can differ from the true value due to various factors.

Carryover Effect

The commonest of problems in crossover design is the carryover effect. In the given example, if the drug A has a carryover effect, the overall result obtained for B may be higher than the true value of B. In sequence 1, the drug A is administered first and the drug B is administered second. The carryover of A may increase the intensity of B's effect. If B is free of carryover effect, in sequence 2, A's effect would not be intensified (Table 13.3).

Table 13.3: Demonstration of the differential carryover effect

Sequence of administration	*Period 1*	*Period 2*
Sequence 1	$A = 6$	$B = 6$
Sequence 2	$B = 4$	$A = 6$

The level of response for the subjects following the sequence 1 of drug administration is different from that of sequence 2. In the first sequence $A - B = 0$, which leads to an erroneous result.

Equal Carryover

In case of equal carryover, effects of both the drugs get amplified in the second period but equal carryover cancels each other. Suppose, the AUC is augmented by 1 unit in the second period. The data will be similar to that of Table 13.4 and result will be unaffected by the carryover.

Table 13.4: Demonstration of the equal carryover effect

Sequence of administration	*Period 1*	*Period 2*
Sequence 1	$A = 6$	$B = 4 + 1$
Sequence 2	$B = 4$	$A = 6 + 1$

$$\frac{[(6-5)-(4-7)]}{2}=2$$

Data Analysis by ANOVA

Prolonged time of the experiment and biovariation factors introduce error in the measurement. The real-life bioequivalence data vary widely and a proper ANOVA is required to interpret such data.

The model used can be depicted by

$$Y_{ijk} = \mu + G_i + S_{ik} + P_j + T_{t\,(ij)} + e_{ijk} \qquad \text{(Eq. 13.3)}$$

Here, Y_{ijk} represents effect of drug observed in subject k, in sequence i and period j.

μ = Overall mean of all observations of all groups.

G_i = Average effect of sequence 'i' (in two-group study the value of 'i' is either 1 or 2). For example, if 1 represents A followed by B and 2 will represent B followed by A.

P_j = Period effect or time effect. In a two-period study the value of j is either 1 or 2.

S_{ik} = Effect observed in subject k in sequence i.

$T_{t\,(ij)}$ = Treatment effect (two treatments A or B).

e_{ijk} = Error associated with subject number k in sequence i and period j.

The source of variations can be categorized as follows.

1. Sequence or the order of treatment may contribute to variations due to carryover effect.
2. The biovariation between subjects; some patients may be more suited to A while others to B.
3. Periods or time effect.
4. Treatment effect (some drugs may be truly different from the other and show different intensity of drug effect).

However, if differential carryover takes place, sequence effects and differential carry over effects get overlapped. So, a proper analysis takes in account all sources of variation.

An example of crossover bioequivalence study for the comparison of two drugs A and B is given in Table 13.5.

The usual ANOVA separates the total sum of squares into four components; subject, sequence, period and treatment. The analysis assumes an absence of differential carry-over effect and the objective of the analysis is to find out whether the treatments are different. A properly done ANOVA should be able to show period effect, detect inter subject variability, difference in treatment and sequence effects.

To account for the variations due to period, two new columns need to be created.

Data for period 1 should contain all results obtained in the first period of the study, irrespective of the type of treatments.

As in each period, 50% of the subjects had taken A and the remaining 50% B, in absence of period effects, data contained under both the periods should be perfectly balanced and sum of the columns should be same.

Table 13.5: Bioequivalence data comparing two groups *A* and *B*

Subject	*Sequence*	*AUC A*	*AUC B*	*Square of AUC (A)*	*Square of AUC (B)*	*Sum of response*	*AUC (A + B) squared*
1	*AB*	25	17	625	289	42	1764
2	*BA*	16	12	256	144	28	784
3	*AB*	14	07	196	49	21	441
4	*AB*	13	04	169	16	17	289
5	*BA*	16	18	256	324	34	1156
6	*BA*	11	09	121	81	20	400
7	*AB*	25	10	625	100	35	1225
8	*BA*	06	15	36	225	21	441
9	*BA*	19	13	361	169	32	1024
10	*AB*	21	11	441	121	32	1024
Sum		166	116	3086	1518		8548
Average		16.6	11.6				

Table 13.6: Bioequivalence data arranged according to period of study

Subject no.	*Period 1*	*Period 2*
1	25	17
2	12	16
3	14	07
4	13	04
5	18	16
6	09	11
7	25	10
8	15	06
9	13	19
10	21	11
Total = 10	165	117
Mean	16.5	11.7

ΣX_t = sum of all observations (t represents total) = 282.

ΣX_A = sum of all observations in formulation A = 166.

ΣX_B = sum of all observations in formulation B = 116.

ΣP_1 = sum of all observations in period 1 = 165.

ΣP_2 = sum of all observations in period 2 = 117.

ΣX_T^2 = sum of the squared observations.

N_t = number of total observations.

$$CT \text{ (correction term)} = \frac{\Sigma X_t^2}{N_t}.$$

ΣS_i = sum of observations for the subject i.

Total sum of squares = $\Sigma X_t^2 - CT$

$$\frac{\Sigma(\Sigma S_i)^2}{2} - CT = \text{Subject sum of squares.}$$

$$\frac{(\Sigma P_1^2 + \Sigma P_2^2)}{N} - CT = \text{Period sum of squares.}$$

$$\frac{(\Sigma X_A^2 + \Sigma X_B^2)}{N} - CT = \text{Treatment sum of squares.}$$

Error sum of squares = Total SS – Subject SS – Period SS – Treatment SS.

In our example,

$$\Sigma X_t = 282$$
$$\Sigma X_A = 166$$
$$\Sigma X_B = 116$$
$$\Sigma P_1 = \text{(from Table 13.6)} = 165$$
$$\Sigma P_2 = \text{(from Table 13.6)} = 117$$
$$\Sigma X_T^2 = 4604$$
$$N_t = \text{Number of total observations} = 10 \times 2 = 20$$

$$CT \text{ (correction term)} = \frac{\Sigma X_t^2}{N_t} = \frac{282^2}{20} = 3976.2$$

$$\Sigma S_i = \text{Sum of observation for the subject } i$$

Total sum of squares = $TSS = \Sigma X_T^2 - CT = 4604 - 3976.2 = 627.8$

Subject sum of squares

$$= \frac{(42^2 + 28^2 + 21^2 + 17^2 + 34^2 + 20^2 + 35^2 + 21^2 + 32^2 + 32^2)}{2}$$

$$\frac{8548}{2} - 3976.2 = 297.8$$

$$\text{Period sum of squares} = \frac{(117^2 + 165^2)}{10} - CT = 4091.4 - 3976.2 = 115.2$$

$$\text{Treatment sum of squares} = \frac{166^2 + 116^2}{10} - CT = 4101.2 - 3976.2 = 125$$

Error sum of squares = Total SS – Subject SS – Period SS – Treatment SS

$627.8 - 297.8 - 115.3 - 125 = 89.8$

Total number of patients is 10; degree of freedom 9

Number of treatments 2; degree of freedom 1

Number of sequences 2; degree of freedom 1

Number of periods 2; degree of freedom 1

Degree of freedom in calculation errors = $N_1 + N_2 - 2$

Where N_1 and N_2 represent number of subjects in each sequence, i.e. 5 + 5 – 2 = 8 (Table 13.7).

Table 13.7: Analysis of variance table for the crossover bioequivalence study of AUC

Source	*d.f.*	*Sum of square*	*Mean sum of squares*	*P*
Subjects	9	297.8	33.08	$F(9/8) = 2.94$
Period	1	115.2	115.2	$F(1/8) = 10.26$*
Treatment	1	125.0	125.0	$F(1/8) = 11.14$*
Error	8	89.8	11.2	

* Indicates $P < 0.05$

The basic assumption of the analysis was absence of carryover effect and hence, the above analysis has not taken into consideration the carryover effect. Any difference due to carryover was merged with the variability of the subjects.

To analyze whether a carryover effect is there or not, a new table is to be created. This table will arrange data according to the sequence of treatment (Table 13.8).

Table 13.8: Arrangement of data for analysis of sequence effect

Group I (treatment A first, B second)				*Group II (treatment B first, A second)*			
Subjects	*A*	*B*	*A + B*	*Subjects*	*A*	*B*	*A + B*
1	25	17	42	2	12	16	28
3	14	07	21	5	16	18	34
4	13	04	17	6	09	11	20
7	25	10	35	8	15	06	21
10	21	11	32	0	13	19	32
Sum = 5	98	49	147	N = 5	65	70	135

$$\text{Sequence sum of squares} = \frac{(\Sigma\text{group } 1^2)}{N_1} + \frac{(\Sigma\text{group } 2^2)}{N_2} - CT$$

$$\text{i.e. } \frac{147^2 + 135^2}{10} - 3976.2 = 7.2$$

Logic of the test is that both the drugs *A* and *B* have been used by the same set of people. Some had taken *A* at first and some had taken *B* first. If the result is not affected by the order of consumption the total effect of group following sequence 1 should be same as total effect of group following sequence 2.

A proper error term should be calculated for this test by deducting the within group sum of squares from the sequence sum of squares.

$$\frac{1}{2}\ \Sigma\ (\text{Subject total})^2 - CT\ (1) - CT\ (2)$$

CT (1) and *CT* (2) represent the correction term of group 1 and group 2.

$\therefore \quad 4274 - 2160.9 - 1822.5 = 290.6$

$\therefore$ Within group sum of squares has a degree of freedom 8.
So within group mean squares

$$= \frac{290.6}{8} = 36.32$$

$$F\,(1/8) = \frac{290.6}{8} = 36.32 \;= 0.198$$

The ratio is insignificant showing there is no sequence effect.

NONPARAMETRIC STATISTICS

For most of the statistical tests it is assumed data are normally distributed. However, there are situations, when data obtained from a study deviate so much from the normal distribution that the assumption of normal distribution is not valid. When nature of distribution is unknown, statistical tests based on normal distribution cannot be applied. Such data are analyzed by distribution-free or nonparametric statistics. Data, which are normally distributed, can also be analyzed by nonparametric methods.

Assumptions: Some assumptions are required in nonparametric statistics too. Data are considered to be,

(*a*) Independent.

(*b*) Continuous in nature.

Types of data usually analyzed by nonparametric statistics

(*a*) ***Nominal data:*** Data or observations are given a name to indicate different categories, e.g. boy or girl, red or black, etc.

(*b*) ***Ranked data:*** Sometimes, a ranking system is used to classify data according to intensity or measure of magnitude. For example, pain can be represented by the ranking of 1, 2 and 3 to indicate mild, moderate and severe pain.

(*c*) ***Interval or ratio scaled data:*** In this type the magnitude of the two data are spaced apart by a definite interval scale, e.g. age (5 years is smaller than 10 years by a specific measure of time).

Sign Test

Sign test is the simplest of nonparametric test. This test is usually used for comparing paired data. The test is a test of equality of the medians of two comparative groups. While comparing two groups, it is often seen that in some pairs, values of first group are higher whereas in other pairs values in the second group are higher. The pairs are matched and differences between each pair are noted. The differences are then categorized only with regard to the sign of the difference. If positive sign and negative sign occur with same frequency, it indicates that treatments have a similar median. If not, there is likelihood that medians are different for both the tests.

Sign test is based on binomial distribution.

Suppose, two creams *A* and *B* are being compared. If the creams are of different quality, there is a possibility that one of the creams will have higher preference than the other.

If the creams are similar in nature, probability exists that both will be preferred to equal degree. The null hypothesis assumes both the creams are similar and the chance of one cream's being favored is only half.

$$H_0: P = 0.5$$

The method of probability calculation depends on sample size.

1. For a sample size of 1–5, i.e. if the number of comparisons is small, the probabilities of the experimental outcomes can be directly calculated from the binomial expression given in equation 1.13 in Chapter 1, which says,
   The probability of *X* successes in *N* trials is

$$\binom{N}{X} p^X q^{N-X}$$

$$\binom{N}{X} = \frac{N!}{X!(N-X)!}$$

2. If *N* ranges from 6 to 20, number of positive or negative signs needed for significance is given in Appendix 6 for 95% confidence level.
3. If sample sizes are greater than 20, probability is calculated by a normal approximation test.

$$Z = \frac{|P - 0.5| - 1/(2N)}{0.5/\sqrt{N}} \qquad \text{(Eq. 13.4)}$$

Where *P* is the observed proportion and *N* is the sample size. The *Z* value obtained from Eq. 13.4 is compared with the reference *Z* value (Appendix 1) for a given degree of freedom.

$$Z = \frac{|\text{number of } +\text{'s} - \text{number of } -\text{'s}| - \frac{1}{2}}{\sqrt{\text{number of } +\text{'s} - \text{number of } -\text{'s}}}$$

Sign test is elementary in nature. Yet it gives an idea whether two groups are likely to be different. Given below is an example of the sign test used for comparison of two groups.

The data above can also be analyzed by more sophisticated tests like *t* test or ANOVA, But if the distributions of the differences are not normal the analysis should be carried out by sign test.

Table 13.9: Comparison of two formulations *A* and *B* for peak plasma conc. (C_{max} μg/ml)

Subject	*Peak. conc. (A)*	*Peak conc. (B)*	*Difference (A – B)*
1	6.0	6.8	−0.8
2	7.0	6.5	+0.5
3	5.8	5.5	+0.3
4	6.0	7.2	−1.2
5	10.0	7.0	+3.0
6	7.5	6.5	+1.0
7	9.0	8.5	+0.5
8	6.8	6.8	0
9	7.1	7.0	+1.0
10	8.1	7.8	+0.3
11	6.5	6.5	0
12	7.3	7.5	−0.2
13	5.5	5.4	+0.1
14	6.0	6.2	−0.2

The procedure can be divided into the following steps:

Step 1: Decision

The sample size is 14. So the table of significance in Appendix 6 is to be used. If more than 20, we would have carried out a Z test as Eq. 13.4.

Step 2: Counting of Signs

Of the 14 samples, 8 have positive sign and two 0 (ties) and 4 have negative sign.

Step 3: Determination of N (Sample Size)

Note that sample size excludes ties. If total number of subjects is 22 and one subject showed same result for the formulations N should be 21 and not 22.

Here, the sample size becomes 14 – 2 = 12.

Step 4: Comparison with the Value given in the Probability Table

Appendix 6 shows out of 12 subjects at 5% level, 10 subjects should have same sign for the formulations to be significantly different. Here, only 8 differences have positive sign. So formulations are not basically different.

Wilcoxon's Signed Rank Test

Wilcoxon's test is a more sensitive nonparametric test than the sign test. In sign test magnitudes of the difference between the paired responses are ignored. In Wilcoxon's signed rank test the magnitudes of the difference between the responses is taken into consideration and hence, it is more powerful test.

Assumptions: The distributions of the treatments are assumed to be symmetrical. To explain this test, again we will use the data given in Table 13.9.

The calculation will be divided into several steps.

Step 1: Initial calculations are same as in sign test. We calculate the difference and its sign.

Step 2: The subjects, who exactly showed equal response, are excluded. The differences of the untied pairs are ranked in order of magnitude disregarding the sign.

Step 3: Differences of equal magnitudes are clubbed together and given a common rank, i.e. an average rank for equal difference.

Step 4: The ranks are reassigned signs.

Step 5: Summation of the positive signs and negative signs.

Step 6: Comparison of the results with the values in Appendix 8 to decide whether the difference is significant.

Examining the data in Table 13.9, we see subjects 8 and 11 had shown exactly equal response. So, they are excluded and the sample size is reduced to 12.

In step 2 the differences are ranked on the basis of the magnitude (Table 13.10 column 3). The smallest difference was observed in subject number 13 and the value is 0.1. So, it gets the first rank. Subjects 14 and 12 show the next higher difference. So, they are assigned 2nd and 3rd ranks. While assigning rank we disregard the sign. So, a negative sign can get 2nd or a positive sign can get 3rd rank or vice versa. Subjects 10 and 3 have the next higher difference, i.e. 0.3 and get ranks 4 and 5. Similarly, other differences are ranked.

Table 13.10: Assignment of ranking for Wilcoxon's signed rank test (Datum is taken from Table 13.9)

Subjects	*Difference*	*Rank*	*Assigned rank*	*Assigned rank with sign*
13	+0.1	1	1.0	+1
14	−0.2	2	2.5	−2.5
12	−0.2	3	2.5	−2.5
10	+0.3	4	4.5	+4.5
3	+0.3	5	4.5	+4.5
7	+0.5	6	6.5	+6.5
2	+0.5	7	6.5	+6.5
1	−0.8	8	8.0	−8.0
9	+1	9	9.5	+9.5
6	+1	10	9.5	+9.5
4	−1.2	11	11	−11
5	+3	12	12	+12

In step 3 the ranks of the subjects having similar differences are averaged and disregarding the sign they are given common rank. For example, only one subject has shown a difference 0.1. So, this group consists of only 1 subject. Hence, the initial rank assigned to this subject is same as the averaged rank, i.e. 1.

Two subjects had shown a difference 0.2 and had ranks 2 and 3.

Average of 2 and 3 = (2 + 3)/2 = 2.5 which is the common assigned rank for subject 12 and 14. Column 4 of Table 13.10 shows the assigned ranks of all differences.

Step 4 shows reassignment of the sign to the ranks. The original signs are brought back in column 5.

In step 5 ranks with positive sign and negative sign are summed (Table 13.11).

Table 13.11: Positive and negative assigned ranks of the subjects

Ranks with positive sign	*Ranks with negative sign*
1	2.5
4.5	2.5
4.5	8.0
6.5	11
6.5	
9.5	
9.5	
12	
Sum = 54	Sum = 24

In step 6, comparison is done to find the significance of results. Appendix 7 gives the values of the smaller of two rank sums needed for significance at 5% level. The *N*, i.e. sample size should be taken as, number of pairs, less the number of ties. For significance, the smaller rank sum must be equal to or less than the designated values in Appendix 7.

The value of the smaller rank sum is 24. For a sample size of 12, the smaller rank sum should be equal to or less than 13 to be significantly different at 5% level. So, the two formulations are not significantly different.

BIBLIOGRAPHY

1. Daniel W Wayne, Biostatistics: *A Foundation for Analysis in Health Sciences*, Seventh edition, John Wiley and Sons, 1999.
2. De Muth James E, Basic statistics and pharmaceutical statistical applications, Marcel Dekker, Inc, 1999.
3. Sanford Bolton, *Practical and Clinical Applications*, Third edition, Marcel Dekker, Inc, 1997.

Appendices

1 *Cumulative Normal Distribution*

Cumulative area under the normal distribution (less than or equal to Z):

Z	*Area*	*Z*	*Area*	*Z*	*Area*	*Z*	*Area*
−3.25	0.0006	−1.50	0.0668	0.25	0.5987	2.00	0.9772
−3.20	0.0007	−1.45	0.0735	0.30	0.6179	2.05	0.9798
−3.15	0.0008	−1.40	0.0808	0.35	0.6368	2.10	0.9821
−3.10	0.0010	−1.35	0.0885	0.40	0.6554	2.15	0.9842
−3.05	0.0011	−1.30	0.0968	0.45	0.6736	2.20	0.9861
−3.00	0.0013	−1.25	0.1056	0.50	0.6915	2.25	0.9878
−2.95	0.0016	−1.20	0.1151	0.55	0.7088	2.30	0.9893
−2.90	0.0019	−1.15	0.1251	0.60	0.7257	2.35	0.9906
−2.85	0.0022	−1.10	0.1357	0.65	0.7422	2.40	0.9918
−2.80	0.0026	−1.05	0.1469	0.70	0.7580	2.45	0.9929
−2.75	0.0030	−1.00	0.1587	0.75	0.7734	2.50	0.9938
−2.70	0.0035	−0.95	0.1711	0.80	0.7881	2.55	0.9946
−2.65	0.0040	−0.90	0.1841	0.85	0.8023	2.60	0.9953
−2.60	0.0047	−0.85	0.1977	0.90	0.8159	2.65	0.9960
−2.55	0.0054	−0.80	0.2119	0.95	0.8289	2.70	0.9965
−2.50	0.0062	−0.75	0.2266	1.00	0.8413	2.75	0.9970
−2.45	0.0071	−0.70	0.2420	1.05	0.8531	2.80	0.9974
−2.40	0.0082	−0.65	0.2578	1.10	0.8643	2.85	0.9978
−2.35	0.0094	−0.60	0.2743	1.15	0.8749	2.90	0.9981
−2.30	0.0107	−0.55	0.2912	1.20	0.8849	2.95	0.9984
−2.25	0.0122	−0.50	0.3085	1.25	0.8944	3.00	0.9987
−2.20	0.0139	−0.45	0.3264	1.30	0.9032	3.25	0.9994
−2.15	0.0158	−0.40	0.3446	1.35	0.9115		
−2.10	0.0179	−0.35	0.3632	1.40	0.9192		
−2.05	0.0202	−0.30	0.3821	1.45	0.9265		
−2.00	0.0228	−0.25	0.4013	1.50	0.9332		
−1.95	0.0256	−0.20	0.4207	1.55	0.9394		
−1.90	0.0287	−0.15	0.4404	1.60	0.9452		
−1.85	0.0322	−0.10	0.4602	1.65	0.9505		
−1.80	0.0359	−0.05	0.4801	1.70	0.9554		
−1.75	0.0401	0	0.5000	1.75	0.9599		
−1.70	0.0446	0.05	0.5199	1.80	0.9641		
−1.65	0.0495	0.10	0.5398	1.85	0.9678		
−1.60	0.0548	0.15	0.5596	1.90	0.9713		
−1.55	0.0606	0.20	0.5793	1.95	0.9744		

Z	*Area*
1.282	0.90
1.645	0.95
1.960	0.975
2.326	0.99
2.576	0.995
3.090	0.999

2 t Distributions

Two-sided:	40%	20%	10%	5%	1%
One-sided:	20%	10%	5%	2.5%	0.5%
d.f.	$t_{0.80}$	$t_{0.90}$	$t_{0.95}$	$t_{0.975}$	$t_{0.995}$
1	1.38	3.08	6.31	12.71	63.66
2	1.06	1.89	2.92	4.30	9.92
3	0.98	1.64	2.35	3.18	5.84
4	0.94	1.53	2.13	2.78	4.60
5	0.92	1.48	2.02	2.57	4.03
6	0.91	1.44	1.94	2.45	3.71
7	0.90	1.42	1.89	2.36	3.50
8	0.89	1.40	1.86	2.31	3.36
9	0.88	1.38	1.83	2.26	3.25
10	0.88	1.37	1.81	2.23	3.17
11	0.88	1.36	1.80	2.20	3.11
12	0.87	1.36	1.78	2.18	3.05
13	0.87	1.35	1.77	2.16	3.01
14	0.87	1.35	1.76	2.14	2.98
15	0.87	1.34	1.75	2.13	2.95
16	0.86	1.34	1.75	2.12	2.92
17	0.86	1.33	1.74	2.11	2.90
18	0.86	1.33	1.73	2.10	2.88
19	0.86	1.33	1.73	2.09	2.86
20	0.86	1.33	1.72	2.09	2.85
25	0.86	1.32	1.71	2.06	2.79
30	0.85	1.31	1.70	2.04	2.75
40	0.85	1.30	1.68	2.02	2.70
60	0.85	1.30	1.67	2.00	2.66
120	0.85	1.29	1.66	1.98	2.62
∞	0.84	1.282	1.645	1.96	2.576

3 Upper 5% Values of the F Distribution

Degrees of freedom in denominator	Degrees of freedom in numerator												
	1	*2*	*3*	*4*	*5*	*6*	*7*	*8*	*9*	*10*	*20*	*40*	*Infinity*
1	161	200	216	225	230	234	237	239	241	242	248	251	254
2	18.5	19.0	19.2	19.2	19.3	19.3	19.4	19.4	19.4	19.4	19.4	19.5	19.5
3	10.1	9.55	9.28	9.12	9.01	8.94	8.89	8.85	8.81	8.79	8.66	8.59	8.53
4	7.71	6.94	6.59	6.39	6.26	6.16	6.09	6.04	6.00	5.96	5.80	5.72	5.63
5	6.61	5.79	5.41	5.19	5.05	4.95	4.88	4.82	4.77	4.74	4.56	4.46	4.37
6	5.99	5.14	4.76	4.53	4.39	4.28	4.21	4.15	4.10	4.06	3.87	3.77	3.67
7	5.59	4.74	4.35	4.12	3.79	3.87	3.79	3.73	3.68	3.64	3.44	3.34	3.23
8	5.32	4.46	4.07	3.84	3.69	3.58	3.50	3.44	3.39	3.35	3.15	3.04	2.93
9	5.12	4.26	3.86	3.63	3.48	3.37	3.29	3.23	3.18	3.14	2.94	2.83	2.71
10	4.96	4.10	3.71	3.48	3.33	3.22	3.14	3.07	3.02	2.98	2.77	2.66	2.54
11	4.84	3.98	3.59	3.36	3.20	3.09	3.01	2.95	2.90	2.85	2.65	2.53	2.40
12	4.75	3.89	3.49	3.26	3.11	3.00	2.91	2.85	2.80	2.75	2.54	2.43	2.30
13	4.67	3.81	3.41	3.18	3.03	2.92	2.83	2.77	2.71	2.67	2.46	2.34	2.21
14	4.60	3.74	3.34	3.11	2.96	2.85	2.76	2.70	2.65	2.60	2.39	2.27	2.13
15	4.54	3.68	3.29	3.06	2.90	2.79	2.71	2.64	2.59	2.54	2.33	2.20	2.07
16	4.49	3.63	3.24	3.01	2.85	2.74	2.66	2.59	2.54	2.49	2.28	2.15	2.01
17	4.45	3.59	3.20	2.96	2.81	2.70	2.61	2.55	2.49	2.45	2.23	2.10	1.96
18	4.41	3.55	3.16	2.93	2.77	2.66	2.58	2.51	2.46	2.41	2.19	2.06	1.92
19	4.38	3.52	3.13	2.90	2.74	2.63	2.54	2.48	2.42	2.38	2.16	2.03	1.88
20	4.35	3.49	3.10	2.87	2.71	2.62	2.51	2.45	2.39	2.35	2.12	1.99	1.84
25	4.24	3.39	2.99	2.76	2.60	2.49	2.40	2.34	2.28	2.24	2.01	1.87	1.71
30	4.17	2.21	2.92	2.69	2.53	2.42	2.33	2.27	2.21	2.16	1.93	1.79	1.62
40	4.08	3.23	2.84	2.61	2.45	2.34	2.25	2.18	2.12	2.08	1.84	1.69	1.51
120	3.92	3.07	2.68	2.45	2.29	2.18	2.09	2.02	1.96	1.91	1.66	1.50	1.25
Infinity	3.84	3.00	2.60	2.37	2.21	2.10	2.01	1.94	1.88	1.83	1.57	1.39	1.00

4 Short Table of Upper 1% Values of the F Distribution

Degrees of freedom in denominator	*Degrees of freedom in numerator*								
	1	*2*	*3*	*4*	*5*	*7*	*10*	*15*	*20*
2	98.49	99.00	99.17	99.25	99.30	99.36	99.39	99.44	99.45
3	34.12	30.82	29.46	28.71	28.24	27.67	27.23	26.87	26.69
4	21.20	18.00	16.69	15.98	15.52	14.98	14.54	14.19	14.02
5	16.26	13.27	12.06	11.39	10.97	10.45	10.05	9.72	9.5
6	13.74	10.92	9.78	9.15	8.75	8.26	7.87	7.56	7.40
8	11.26	8.65	7.59	7.01	6.63	6.19	5.82	5.52	5.36
10	10.04	7.56	6.55	5.99	5.64	5.21	4.85	4.56	4.41
15	8.68	6.36	5.42	4.89	4.56	4.14	3.80	3.52	3.36
20	8.10	5.85	4.94	4.43	4.10	3.70	3.37	3.09	2.94
30	7.56	5.39	4.51	4.02	3.70	3.30	2.98	2.70	2.55
40	7.31	5.18	4.31	3.83	3.51	3.12	2.80	2.52	2.37
60	7.08	4.98	4.13	3.65	3.34	2.95	2.63	2.39	2.20
100	6.90	4.82	3.98	3.51	3.20	2.82	2.51	2.22	2.06
Infinity	6.63	4.60	3.78	3.32	3.02	2.64	2.32	2.04	1.87

5 Short Table of Chi-Square Distributions

Probability	*Degrees of freedom*												
	1	*2*	*3*	*4*	*5*	*6*	*7*	*8*	*9*	*10*	*15*	*20*	*30*
0.99	6.63	9.21	11.3	13.3	15.1	16.8	18.5	20.1	21.7	23.2	30.6	37.6	50.9
0.975	5.02	7.38	9.35	11.1	12.8	14.45	16.0	17.5	19.0	20.5	27.5	34.2	47.0
0.95	3.84	5.99	7.81	9.49	11.1	12.6	14.1	15.5	16.9	18.3	25.0	31.4	43.8
0.90	2.71	4.61	6.25	7.78	9.24	10.6	12.0	13.4	14.7	16.0	22.3	28.4	40.3

6 Number of Positive or Negative Signs Needed for Significance for the Sign Test

Sample size	*Number of positive or negative signs for significance**	
	5% level	*1% level*
6	6	–
7	7	–
8	8	8
9	8	9
10	9	10
11	10	11
12	10	11
13	11	12
14	12	13
15	12	13
16	13	14
17	13	15
18	14	15
19	15	16
20	15	17

* This is a two-sided test. Choose positive or negative sign, whichever is larger.

7 Values Leading to Significance for the Wilcoxon Signed Rank Test (Two-Sided Test)

Sample size, N	*5% level**	*1% level*
6	0	—
7	2	—
8	3	0
9	5	1
10	8	3
11	10	5
12	13	7
13	17	10
14	21	13
15	25	16
16	30	19
17	35	23
18	40	28
19	46	32
20	52	37

* If the smaller rank sum is less than or equal to the table value, the comparative groups are different at the indicated level of significance.

8 Random Numbers

44	17	50	92	09	79	27	71	05	07	76	21	95	93	04
83	50	39	13	89	83	45	72	40	94	78	62	93	55	62
28	79	77	81	43	04	54	23	14	80	49	98	32	70	27
55	29	62	11	00	62	65	76	31	83	08	22	02	35	53
88	93	30	81	50	24	43	07	88	45	96	24	60	78	89
46	00	76	13	83	31	98	15	30	74	17	76	73	31	40
99	05	78	83	75	79	52	47	39	12	70	33	42	30	45
24	88	59	45	16	73	64	63	03	16	04	43	81	66	97
14	90	27	33	43	46	37	68	94	35	12	72	70	43	54
50	27	98	87	19	20	15	73	00	94	52	85	80	22	26
55	47	03	77	04	44	22	78	84	26	04	33	46	09	52
59	29	97	68	60	71	91	38	67	54	13	58	18	24	76
48	55	90	65	72	96	57	69	36	10	96	46	92	42	45
66	37	32	20	30	77	84	57	03	29	10	45	65	04	26
68	49	69	10	82	53	75	91	93	30	34	25	20	57	27
83	62	64	11	12	67	19	00	71	74	60	47	21	92	86
06	90	91	47	68	25	49	33	74	02	16	29	35	65	16
33	23	97	78	26	78	26	45	40	19	61	29	33	73	09
47	15	40	15	02	82	06	93	20	01	67	38	02	37	90
79	65	14	62	16	34	96	02	75	82	46	75	43	89	36

Index

C

D

M

N

O

P

Q

R

S

T

U

V